HATHA YOGA
The Hidden Language

HATHA YOGA

The Hidden Language

Symbols, Secrets, and Metaphor

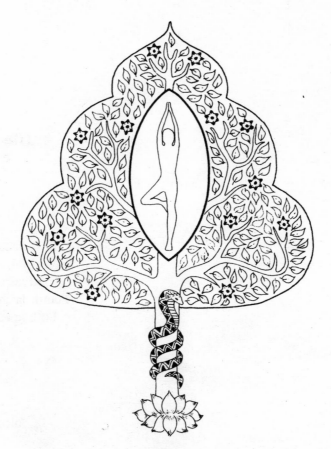

JAICO PUBLISHING HOUSE

MUMBAI • DELHI • BANGALORE • HYDERABAD
KOLKATA • CHENNAI • AHMEDABAD

Published in arrangement with :
Timeless books
Box 160
Porthill, ID 83853

HATHA YOGA
(The Hidden Language)
ISBN 81-7224-120-8

First Jaico Impression : 1993
Second Jaico Impression : 1996
Third Jaico Impression : 1998
Fourth Jaico Impression : 2002
Fifth Jaico Impression : 2003

Published by:
Jaico Publishing House
121, M.G. Road,
Mumbai-400 023

Printed by :
Gayatri Offset Press
A-66, Sector-2, Noida-201301

DEDICATED . . .

To Swami Sivananda Saraswati, my Guru and "Spiritual Mother." Gurudev Sivananda's true greatness of character is a beacon of Light and compassion in an age of darkness. May his Light be a blessing to all.

acknowledgements

I would like to express my appreciation to all those who have helped to prepare this book for publication. My special thanks go to Bob Frager and Arthur Hastings of the Institute for Transpersonal Psychology for their support, to Rita Foran and Margaret Gray for their skilled editing, and to Dawn Spickler for her careful research into many aspects of symbolism. I also wish to mention Margaret White for her artistic contribution, Linda Pelton for designing the book, and Linda Anne Seville for the photographic work.

My gratitude goes to Mr. B.K.S. Iyengar for his encouragement as the manuscript took shape, and for the use of quotations from his book, *Sparks of Divinity*.

table of contents

STRUCTURES

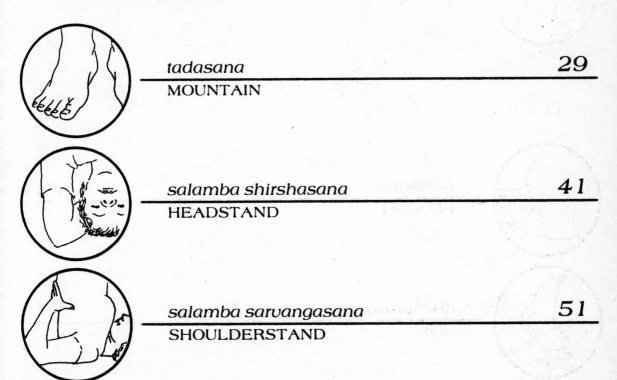

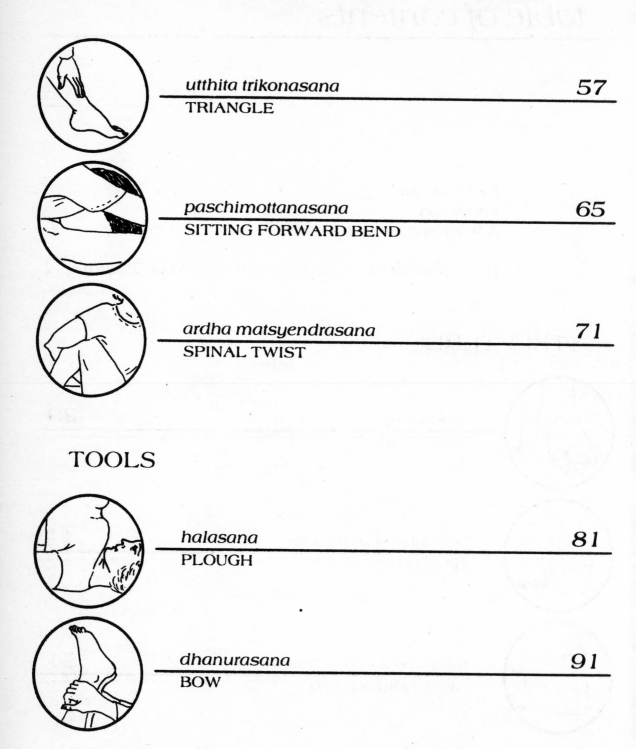

PLANTS

FISH, REPTILES, INSECTS

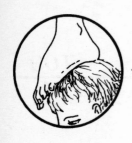
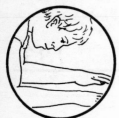
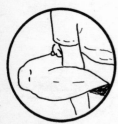
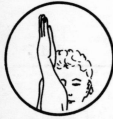
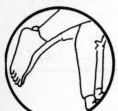

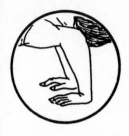
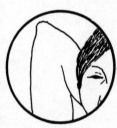
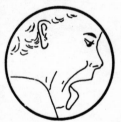
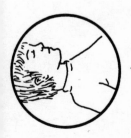

RAMAMANI IYENGAR MEMORIAL YOGA INSTITUTE

1107-B/1, SHIVAJINAGAR, PUNE 411 016, (INDIA).

Date   24-11-1985

Dear Swami Radha,

It was kind of you to have sent me *Hatha Yoga: The Hidden Language* by your good self.

I went through the manuscript. It is a good way of explaining the asanas symbolically so that each asana prepares the sadhaka's mind to see the asana in its true perspective.

Unfortunately, Hatha Yoga is often misunderstood, even by intellectuals, philosophers, saints, and many yogis. It is not just physical Yoga. If *Hatha* is taken as a single word, it conveys the meaning of "The Science of Will." If they are taken separately, then *ha* stands for Sun and *tha* stands for Moon. Many have given the physiological meaning as Suryanadi and Chandranadi—*Surya* for sympathetic nerves, *Chandra* for parasympathetic nerves, and *sushumna* for the central or electrical nervous system.

If the word *Hatha* is considered psychologically and philosophically, it conveys that Sun which never fades and which stands for *atma* (soul). Atma is ever alert, divine, and dynamic. The Chandra stands for the Moon. The Moon being the reflected light of the Sun, consciousness (tha) is the reflected light of the soul. Knowing and realising it, is Hatha Yoga.

Hatha Yoga teaches us to use the body as the bow, asana as the arrow, and the soul as the target. It is a fact that not one has realised the soul without using the body, the mind, the intelligence, and the consciousness (which are all parts of nature) as a means to realise it. When they are cultivated, they become refined and merge in the soul. This is divine absorption, the effect of Hatha Yoga.

In Part I of the *Hatha Pradipika*, the importance of ethical discipline to Hatha Yoga has also been emphasised. As these ethical disciplines were then in vogue, the text did not have to elaborate upon them.

I am glad that you have given thought as to how the Yoga sadhakas can do the asanas by beginning with connective action and ending with reflection, contemplation, and absorption. I hope your work will help to build the bridge between body, mind, and soul, so that later these three compartmental attentions can transform into a single attention for the transfiguration of the true self.

With regards,

B.K.S. Iyengar

preface

Wʜᴇɴ ᴍᴏꜱᴛ ᴘᴇᴏᴘʟᴇ in the West think of Yoga, they think of yoga asanas or postures. They think of them as a form of exercise. Too often, even with experienced students, the asanas are practised with this thought in mind. Swami Radha warns us that there are also yoga teachers who teach asanas without an understanding of their real nature and purpose. Asanas are a devotional practice which, like all spiritual practices, bring us closer to an understanding of the truth.

The most common reason students give for taking a yoga asana class is that they are seeking relief from some musculoskeletal problem, or that they want to learn how to relax. Few people express an interest in the spiritual aspects—in the beginning. However, those who stay with the practice inevitably begin to make certain discoveries. First they often do feel better physically. They begin to breathe and move more freely. Their state of mind changes, their concentration improves, and they become more alert, more fully alive. And then something else begins to emerge: the sense that while this is a very desirable state of affairs, there is something more. The student begins to get glimpses of an aspect of self beyond the physical, mental, emotional levels—a glimpse of the truth about this entity called "myself."

Each asana affords certain physical, physiological, and psychological benefits. Beyond this there also lies a mystical or spiritual meaning. Each asana creates a certain meditative state of mind. But why *these* positions? Why *these* names?

One reason for these postures is that they are anatomically correct, and when properly practised utilize the full and natural range of movement of the human body. They promote efficient functioning of the internal organs, balance the sympathetic and parasympathetic nervous systems, and create an optimum state of health and well-being for each individual to fulfill their own destiny.

The asanas are also symbols. When I practise them I make a symbolic gesture with my body, mind, and breath, and my experience builds a bridge between these aspects of myself and the source of energy which creates and sustains them.

One group of asanas is named after animals, some are geometric structures, some are universal symbols; many arise from ancient myths. In *A Dictionary of Symbols,* J. E. Cirlot says, "Symbolism was an essential part of the ancient art of the Orient and of the medieval tradition in the West. It has been lately revived in the study of the unconscious, both directly in the field of dreams, visions, and psycho-analysis and indirectly in art and poetry."

Yoga is an art and the asanas are a poetic expression of that art—symbols which can unlock the truth and lead us toward the Light. In this book, with her usual thoroughness and insight, Swami Radha has presented another valuable tool for serious students of Yoga who wish to understand the symbolic language of asanas and how to express it, body and soul, in their practice.

Shirley Daventry French
Founder, Victoria Yoga Centre
Victoria, British Columbia

a word from the author

HATHA YOGA PLAYS an important part in the development of a human being. It leads to an exploration of the potential of the body, working in harmony with the mind, to bring the seeker into closer contact with the Higher Self. This book is for those who, in practicing Hatha Yoga, want to find a deeper meaning in the asanas. The meaning is there, psychologically and spiritually, and one can now begin to look at the postures as symbols and find in them an unsuspected significance.

The asanas are named in groups: animals, plants, birds, structures. The name of the asana is the place to begin looking for its symbolic meaning. For example: *Mountain*—strong, massive, immovable, insurmountable, high. What have mountains meant to peoples of different cultures? What does mountain mean to me? My inner strength, my immovability (stubbornness?), my strivings, my insurmountable obstacles, my lofty ideals? As I stand in this posture and view it as a symbol, my struggles to reach the top, the stretching of my body and the effort of my muscles help me to see different aspects of myself and gain new insights.

The symbolic meaning of the name from the myths and traditions of different countries helps to bring an understanding of the universality of the symbol and, by exploring less familiar interpretations, it is possible to broaden the limits of our own understanding.

The body is the instrument through which we act out our desires and exercise our will. Bringing the body under control through the discipline of Hatha Yoga and reflection on the symbolic meaning of the asanas, will also help to bring the mind and emotions under control.

As an asana is perfected through practice, at a certain stage it becomes spiritual, a *mudra*. The word *mudra* means "a seal, a sealing posture." The royal houses and nobility use seals to signify their position and authenticity. In ancient times the seal was the confirmation of the sender of a message. The human body is also a seal. We have to discover what is sealed up, what is the secret behind the seal. To do that we must begin the process of deciphering what the body conveys.

What is discovered from the practice of asanas becomes an enormous source of energy and inspiration to understand more. We are to ourselves like a book with seven seals; we don't know who we really are, what we are, and we rarely ask this question. We go through life with all the aches and pains, mentally and emotionally, all the frustrations, and we feel a helpless victim of all these energies when in actuality we have not yet accepted that we are the masters of our own destiny.

In the Eastern tradition you are a discoverer, an adventurer, and you become your own laboratory, making your own investigations. It is up to each person to think intuitively, to investigate, to inquire, because the yoga teacher will not take the joy and pleasure of discovery from a student. Beyond the spoken word lies intuitive listening. The mystical message in Hatha Yoga must be understood by intuitive perception. An excellent way to develop this is by taking time to reflect.

In due time one becomes aware that the practice of Hatha Yoga is not limited to the physical. It begins there because human awareness is, in the beginning, physical. The effect of the practice of asanas on the central nervous system must be given serious attention. Through continued practice there will be a slow adjustment and development, and greater awareness of the voluntary and involuntary nervous systems will come about. All yoga postures tend to normalize the functions of the entire organism and, therefore, affect the activity of the glands and the different organs, as well as the nervous system and thus the mind. The practice of Yoga will lead to increasing self-mastery, and it will become obvious that this is a formidable power.

Self-mastery means control of the mind and all its functions, including speech. The implications of speech are so important in the yogic process that it is symbolized by a special goddess, the Devi of Speech. She is an essential part of the Kundalini Yoga system, which includes Hatha Yoga, and she is often incorporated into the sections of this book, in the lists of words to be investigated by the individual and used as a basis for personal expansion of the symbols.

In the ancient Yogic Teachings there is a story of the spiritual search of a king named Milinda, who sought far and wide to find a sage wise enough to answer his questions. At last the venerable Nagasena came to him, and the conversations between the two are widely quoted in this book as they tell succinctly the lessons to be learned from the animals whose names have been given to some of the yoga asanas.*

*The conversations between King Milinda and Nagasena are published in *Sacred Books of the East,* vols. 35 and 36.

YOGA PSYCHOLOGY & YOGA THERAPY

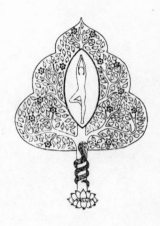

introduction

YOGA PSYCHOLOGY & YOGA THERAPY

EVERY MAN AND WOMAN is a bridge between two worlds, the material and the mental. The body is the material tangible side, subject to its own laws; the mind, which uses the body as a tool of expression (frequently violating the physical laws), has its own realm of time and space where it roams about, often undirected or misdirected. The body is material—the bones, muscles, blood, and everything that makes up the cells. The brain, too, is material. The mind, however, is immaterial and intangible; we can only become aware of it through its manifestation in thought and other functions.

Two worlds: body and mind

All of our five senses, located in the body, act as input and output instruments of perception. Through our senses we experience the world around us (input); mind is the interpreter of all those experiences and, in turn, stimulates the senses to action (output). There is often more input through the senses than mind and emotions can handle. When the output of action does not balance with the input, the result can range from mild disaster to catastrophe. Hatha Yoga in its various aspects is a means to bring the input-output into balance, and to obtain a new understanding of the body as a tool that can function much beyond the limitations usually determined by our beliefs and attitudes.

Input and output through the senses

The human being functions in polarity and this is expressed in the meaning of the word *Hatha*. *Ha* means "the sun, heat, light, energy, creativity, activity, passion, positive," and *tha* means "the moon, cool, reflective, receptive, negative." The terms *positive* and *negative* also refer to the electrical-chemical charge of the body, the right side being positively charged and the left negatively. We are dealing here with two extremes: heat and cold, activity and inactivity, positive and

Ha and tha

negative. The mind also has its own polarities. Life is mainly of such a nature; we move from one extreme to the other. This takes place because of preconceived ideas and a wide range of set opinions and assumptions. The ultimate goal of yogic practices is to be in the center.

YOGA AND THE WHOLE PERSON

Balancing polarities

The meaning of *Yoga* is "union," the bringing together of the various polarities within, in order to reach a state of balance and transcend our limited vision. But Truth is approached by degrees. We have first to know the truth about ourselves. We have learned to cover up our many fears very well. In Hatha Yoga we confront our fears as well as our potentials by balancing attention between the body and the mind; for example, a person who has a neck and shoulders as unyielding as a piece of steel is probably unyielding in daily life. Asanas might loosen up the neck and shoulders temporarily, but becoming aware of the psychological implications will help to make the change more permanent. By observing and dealing with the mental-emotional processes, awareness and understanding are increased. Reverence for one's body, as for all life, is an antidote to abuse and violence. When the relatedness of the physical and the mental is better understood, the mind can function as its own therapist by shifting focus, with reprogramming as the intended choice.

Body and mind interconnected

Through the practice of asanas, students will become aware of stress in the body and, by the use of their own minds, discover many of their problems. Changes can then be made in life by a conscious decision on the basis of will and self-analysis. The inability to cope with stress, and the sense of helplessness and hopelessness that many people experience, can be counteracted by recognizing the options and applying the power of choice.

Power of choice

Unfortunately, in the West, Yoga of any type has often been confused in the lay person's mind with Eastern religions or

4.

cults. Yoga is not a religion, although its practice is used by many religions to help their followers. The physical, psychological, and spiritual aspects are of utmost importance and have always been the basis on which the various Yogas, Kundalini and Hatha specifically, have been built to achieve the harmonious development of human beings. It is, however, essential to have some understanding of the culture[1] from which Yoga has sprung if one intends to work with it; otherwise the "spirit" will be missed and, as a result, more harm than good may be done.

Understanding Eastern culture

Hatha Yoga is a human science that takes into consideration bodily pains, poor posture, faulty breathing, and incorrect walking, teaching greater awareness of the body as a whole, without separating it from the mind and the influences of all the senses. It is not a separate system from Kundalini; each has its own complexities. Since Yoga has become known in the West, the Kundalini system[2] has been compartmentalized, often beyond recognition. This reductionist view has prevented the achievement of the promised results. Kundalini has many branches, like a tree, and Hatha Yoga is one of them. In this presentation Hatha Yoga is singled out to obtain a clearer understanding at a very basic level so that the entire system can be better appreciated.

Kundalini system

However, because human beings are so complex, various branches of Yoga must be practiced in proper combination to help people become harmonious beings beyond the fulfillment of their immediate needs; and it takes time for the whole picture to emerge. It would be a mistake to practice Hatha Yoga, limiting it to the physical aspects only, and leave out other branches of the tree of life such as Bhakti Yoga, Jnana Yoga, or Raja Yoga. (The *Bhagavad Gita* mentions eighteen different Yogas.) Mantra Yoga,[3] which is part of Bhakti, the Yoga of devotion, uses repetition of the sacred sound or the Divine Name. Aspirants will often receive from their Guru (teacher) a Mantra to be practiced together with the asanas. If the mind has a higher focus such as Mantra while one is in an asana, the benefit to the body will be greater, and adverse

Branches of Yoga

Mantra

psychological characteristics will become evident through the symbolism of the postures themselves.

The asanas named after beasts, birds, reptiles, and so on, do not refer to a lower-than-the-human kingdom whose postural patterns they try to imitate. They are meant to remind one that the world is a place in which many living creatures have their existence. All life is sacred.

Learning from
animals

B.K.S. Iyengar, who has developed a rigorous and demanding yoga system, has grouped the asanas to demonstrate particular qualities of a species, with the explanation that one has to pay reverence to each, and that we should never be too proud to learn from their characteristics. This is also verified in the delightful discussions between King Milinda and the sage Nagasena,[4] which show clearly that with the right attitudes of modesty, sincerity, and humility one can learn from every encounter.

Interdependency of
body and mind

Asanas are a discipline of the body, but they are not without an effect on the mind; and, in turn, the mind affects the body. This interdependency needs to be considered. Individuals must accept full responsiblity for their mental-emotional reactions, as well as for the development of their body. This is emphasized in the traditional Hatha Yoga texts. All teachers have stressed the need for a good balance in order to become a well-developed person.

In writing this book, my intention is to offer to the ordinary individual what is usually only available to the scholar or devotee of a knowledgeable Master. Many Westerners, even those who teach the asanas, are not aware of the very subtle influences these body postures have on the mind, emotions,

Role of the Guru

and central nervous system. In fact, the physiological and psychological influences are little understood by most modern yoga teachers because those finer points, never limited to just physical flexibility or health, are only given by the Guru directly to the devotee. Most people who practice just Hatha Yoga never truly become devotees of a Guru, and thereby miss the wealth that could be theirs. Because their focus is on the body, they not only overlook these influences, but are unaware of the hidden effects they exert.[5] Neither does the teacher realize his or her impact in the classroom. When attention is focused on the body in order to do the posture, another part of the mind is influenced by the instructor's words, such as in Paschimottanasana: "Sit straight; keep your spine straight; bend from the hips; inhale—stretch forward; exhale—relax into the posture." It is very important that the words used are carefully chosen for positive effects.

Importance of speech in teaching

Hatha Yoga teachers will find that the students in their classes who have few problems will have a good start for their personal development. But there may also be those who are having serious emotional difficulties, and they do not belong in the class. They should be referred to other professionals who accept Yoga as an alternative tool. This kind of respect and cooperation helps to bridge the Eastern-Western approaches, benefiting all concerned.

Students with serious emotional problems

PSYCHOLOGY EAST AND WEST

Body, mind, and spirit have, in the West, been separated into distinct areas as required by our scientific systems, and put into traditionally acceptable structures with little consideration for the whole human being. Only recently have different ways been sought and explored. The new holistic health movement has opened the gateway to the royal road of Yoga, leading to physical, mental-emotional, and spiritual harmony.

Body, mind, and spirit

A swami with a mind bent on scientific proof, Kuvalaya-nanda, who was a member of the Central Health Education Bureau in New Delhi, makes a number of statements that are insightful, especially regarding the use of Yoga and its psychology as therapy. These seem to be in harmony with the Western school of Transpersonal Psychology. That name implies the transcending of the personality and its many aspects as one of the basic premises. Swami Kuvalayananda

Yoga Psychology

suggests that it is more important to pay attention to the pattern of developing into the posture, and to observe the psychological implications, than to try to accomplish the posture exactly and thereby miss the purpose of the asana, namely, the discovery of the physical obstacles that have their root in the personality make-up.

Gymnastics and asanas

He also emphasizes that the distinction between gymnastics and asanas lies not only in the degree of contraction, but that there is "a) the separate neural basis for each, and b) the tonic interoceptive impulses which [in asanas] are not only more economical of energy, but have a far reaching psycho-physiological bearing on the behavior of man."[6] But even a steady posture, when accomplished, does not resolve itself into a cessation of neuro-muscular activity.

Individual differences taken into account

He clearly points out that asanas have to be performed in a particular way to suit not only the body and mental-emotional temperament of the individual, but also the intelligence and level of understanding. Of course, it has to be remembered that learning in the East is done under the guidance and close observation of a personal Guru. B.K.S. Iyengar is very firm on the point that asanas must be done correctly, according to his precise instructions, and only then will the mental-emotional, and the positive-negative, tendencies come into harmony.

Reflection and awareness essential

These opposite tendencies in the mind can only be brought together by a common denominator: greater awareness in living, more depth—in other words, quality in all areas of personal life. This implies that it is not sufficient to have harmonious breathing while practicing the postures. It will certainly aid but never replace reflection and focus on the qualities one intends to bring into life.

Conquer the mind

"Mind," says Iyengar, "is the king of the senses. One who has conquered his mind, senses and passions, thought and reason, is a king among men. He has Inner Light."[7]

The first step toward this Light is perhaps insight into the need for a psychology that will deal with the rational and irrational, with an external and an internal reality. The intuitive, the symbolic, the poetic, will then point to the source from which happiness and joy grow. The importance of the inner subjective and meditative as well as the introspective capacities, while rejected by many orthodox schools, has always been known by Eastern and by transpersonal psychologists. All experiences are worth remembering, acknowledging, and learning from, even if they are not joyful and aesthetic. The most elevating happenings can be misused by human greediness and selfishness; nevertheless, all factors or capabilities have to be taken into consideration to achieve a healthy balance in the struggle to become an all-round developed, harmonious being.[8]

Learning from all experiences

Most problems lie within the many personalities that make up the overall personality and that play their roles in a fierce competitive way, sometimes even being at war with each other as when we are "of two minds." The discipline of Yoga helps one gradually to transcend those personalities. One may begin with the body and observe "all the rules"—like cleanliness, being in the fresh air, using natural fibers, and even becoming a vegetarian. But unless the intelligence recognizes that pure food does not deliver a pure mind, or putting on a different type of robe does not make one a gentle and loving person, one will find that violence, resentments, and many other compulsive emotions still lurk under all the cover-ups.

Transcending personality aspects

Abraham Maslow, the noted psychologist, has said that a good psychologist must be humble, by which he meant to be understanding, loving, and tender-minded, even if it resulted in being less scientific. He has also seen psychology as impoverished from having been cut off from philosophy.[9] This view is very much in harmony with the psychology of Yoga and the Yogic Teachings. The motivation comes from a sincere heart, a desire to help in any possible way, which is precisely why Yoga is divided into so many different branches to suit the many individual temperaments and their needs. It must be remembered that to learn more about oneself means to learn more

Humility and motivation

YOGA PSYCHOLOGY

about people in general.

In recent years, Western psychology has become bolder and more creative, venturing into new areas. Transpersonal Psychology not only has earnestly tried the road of discovery in spite of sometimes encountering hostility, but also has been cautious and careful to avoid mistakes. Its creativeness and inventiveness, unorthodox at times, has allowed it to become a compassionate, living instrument to meet the needs of people. It has pursued new ideas in order to get results, and afterward mapped out the methods that can be applied by others in the field. Transpersonal Psychology is still open-ended and growing; its aims take it beyond the usual limits of psychology. It is the individual, not the particular line of thought that has been developed by certain scientists, that is the central point. Being realistic is not only to identify with the negative, the misery and failure, but also to see victories and the basically good characteristics that are innate in human nature. These need to be shown on the other side of the scales if a healthy balance is to be achieved. Transpersonal Psychology might be defined, therefore, as a psychology that will lead toward meanings and values that point out the ultimate or the highest as perceived by the individual.[10]

*Bridging Yoga and
Western science*

Elmer and Alyce Green, of the Menninger Foundation, provided for me, as a Westerner trained in the yogic tradition, one of the first bridges between Yoga and the scientific techniques of the West. They are of the opinion that "the development of the totally integrated man, a personal and transpersonal synthesis, is the affirmed goal in modern yogic teaching, but the need for voluntary quieting of mental, emotional, and physiological processes, with an accompanying focus of attention on transpersonal awareness, is not easy for the personal self to accept."[11]

*Self-importance
and selfishness*

The Greens have also expressed the opinion that some people hope to be saved without any effort on their part, expecting simply to make the personal-transpersonal integration into a personal change that excludes dealing with self-importance and selfishness. Many Gurus state that "selfless service will make you Divine." Although it is helpful to know something about the state of Satchitananda, or "resting in one's own Atman," this intellectual perception will not guarantee the realization of one's divinity, while self-less service will indeed grant that recognition. Not only the Vedas, but also sacred texts of other cultures, are full of the need to sacrifice, to forego, or to renounce the fruits of development of personal powers such as siddhis, and to transcend the personality that would like to demonstrate these powers for self-gratification and personal power.

Selfless service and renouncing the fruits

It has been demonstrated through biofeedback, in the work of the Greens and later work done in the West, that it is possible to tell the body what to do by applying will power and strong imaginative desire. The power of concentration and imagination applied to the asanas and what they imply puts the body into a kind of "listening mode." Receptivity overcomes the argumentative mode and makes the body relaxed and receptive to its own messages, without suggestion or hypnosis. There are variances in how to tell the body, depending on the type of mind and temperament. But if an urgent state of illness demands quick help, one may resort to the power of suggestion and hypnosis.

Putting the body into a listening mode

The power of self-hypnosis (the process by which one responds to repeated suggestions within one's own mind) has come into wide application by the Simonton group, some of whose patients have used the terms *the enemies* and *the good knights* to mobilize their bodies against cancer. The enemies are the cancer cells that are fought by the good knights—the healthy cells. In Yoga spiritual aspects would be included. The power of suggestion would not be limited to good and bad, black and white, but rather the positive forces would be turned into rays of Light in which anything detrimental would dissolve.

Dissolving illness in Light

From time to time the limitations that come from tradition and established concepts have to be loosened and the dead wood be cut out to give room for new growth. Otto Rank, considered by some to be the most brilliant of Freud's pupils, was convinced that humans have always lived beyond the traditional in the irrational, and that by accepting the irrational, vital human values were rediscovered. In recent times medicine has taken this view into account, whereas traditionally, medicine neglected to look at the whole person. Healing is dependent not only on diagnostic arts but also on the healing reserves of the body being summoned. The controversy between philosophical and theoretical medical healing shows some differences still exist. Ill persons have to be seen in their social and cultural setting; analysis of language use, of personal symbolism, and of the structure of the body can be useful.

The body's healing reserves

Western psychology has dealt extensively with the subject of pain, and at least one author[12] has associated the positive management of pain with imagination. In the Kundalini system, the third chakra (Manipura), which controls emotions and feelings, carefully examines pain, specifically to distinguish what is self-inflicted because of wrong attitudes and uncultivated imagination. In such an examination, various aspects of pain will emerge, and it is wise to write them down and take them one by one for further scrutiny. Such involvement with thinking about them brings new insights that help to get to the root of the problem so that it can be overcome. Of course, if pain of any type persists, then the necessary medical help should be sought. A therapist also may ease mental-emotional distress. Teamwork, having a variety of tools available, can aid in the process of healing.

Pain

SYMBOLISM AND SPEECH

Imagination and attitudes are shaped by the words we use. The repetition in the mind of words and phrases plays a large part in the state of health of body or mind. In the West the emphasis has been on body, mind, and spirit, whereas the triad in the East is body, mind, and speech, because speech is recognized as man's greatest achievement. The individual has to deal

Body, mind, and speech

directly with the interaction between body, mind, and speech, and their various interdependencies. Without careful work the transcendence of the many personality aspects will be extremely difficult, if not impossible. Symbolism is very helpful for understanding these complexities; for example, in doing Garudasana one's own aggressiveness may become apparent. The gentle way of reflecting on symbolism allows for an individual pace without direct confrontation within oneself or with others. Without confrontation, insights arise that eliminate the need for self-defence and self-justification.

Reflecting on symbolism

The interactions between body and mind can be clearly experienced, but speech, the mouthpiece of both, will be able to interact with them effectively only when skillfully used. Awareness of the intonation of the voice, and control of emotions and breath, focus the power of speech and make the words fly like an arrow to their target. Mantra Yoga, which has already been mentioned, is a means of lifting speech from the daily chatter to a higher level. The repetition of a sacred word or holy name will help to diminish careless thinking and speech. Sometimes a dialogue with the Divine, or thoughts written in a spiritual diary, will bring greater clarity and skill of expression.

Focusing the power of speech

Mantra is connected with the power of speech, in some sacred texts called the Devi of Speech. Speech has a psychological, and sometimes even hypnotic, impact on the mind. The power of the spoken word is most clearly shown in the practice of Mantra. Even if one does not know the meaning of the words, the effect is apparent. The composition of the words of Mantras as sounds is the power of creation—the power of inspiration and illumination. The letters of the Sanskrit (Indian) alphabet are on the petals of the chakras of the Kundalini system, indicating the importance that is given to the inner experience of language.[13] Letters and words are the symbols in everyday life that give outward expression to our thoughts and ideas.

Power of Mantra

At first a symbol is recognized only on a certain level; then it moves to other levels, according to the grasp of the user.

Emotions experienced in the body are forces whose effect on either body or mind is often not understood. The symbolism that is used in the idioms and expressions of daily language plays a much larger part in life than is usually acknowledged; it can help individuals to understand their unconscious. Through reflection one can see that ideas are themselves formless, even though the symbol gives them form. If attachments are deeply rooted, seeing them in symbolic form can help to loosen them.

The use of symbols illustrates the dependence, interdependence, and interaction between the body and the mind. An example of how this can be useful is perhaps best demonstrated by looking at the way sound or melody is created. Melody depends on:

a) the instrument, the flute
b) air/breath
c) the flute player

None of these by itself can produce melody or sound, but each depends upon the interaction with the others.

In the practice of the asanas, the interconnection of body, mind, and speech is a little more complex. Speech is more than the exchange of words with others; it is also talking to oneself, be it audibly or just in the mind. In the learning of each asana there will also be a learning of the dependence, interdependence, and interaction related to body, mind, and speech.

INVESTIGATING THE MIND

The mind is an elusive tool for investigating itself, but it is the only tool there is. A good starting point in investigating the mind is to list its various functions, see how they are already reflected in the emotions, and realize that a conscious effort has to be made to separate the mental function and the emotional implications in order to clearly see. It takes time to discover patterns of mind and patterns of emotions. The interplay of these activities is muddled and points to the need to achieve discriminative awareness. It is astonishing to see how easily one can be lost in mind-created distortions and pain.

Concentration—that is, focusing on something—depends largely on the thinking process, and the method by which the individual attempts to concentrate. Some people see in their mind's eye the image of a cat when the word *cat* is pronounced; we may call them concrete thinkers. Other people will "see" the letters c-a-t; we may call them abstract thinkers. This rather oversimplified distinction serves our purpose for now. There are people whose thinking is so fast or so vague that they cannot say either way. In this case, it may be helpful to practice "watching the mind"[14] in conjunction with the practice of postures.

Concentration

The mind is like a wild horse. It takes continuous effort to keep it quiet and free from distractions for any period of time. Psychological obstacles will push their way with all their might to get back into a dominant position. They will fight for the "right" that they have been granted for a lifetime. It is best to quickly give the mind some activity to keep it reined in: "What does a tortoise mean to me?" List the inpouring thoughts in a notebook for later reference; for example, a tortoise is slow-moving, withdraws into its shell; hard shell, soft body, ungainly, beautiful patterns on its shell. If these words are understood as symbols for something else, one can see their relatedness to individual problems.

Giving the mind a focus

It becomes more and more obvious how thoughts have their own effects on the body and the body, in turn, affects the mind. The psychology of Yoga demands that all intrusions from mind's interpretation of the input from the senses be dealt with in order to lay a solid foundation of self-development on which to build new experience. The process of clarification of words used aloud as well as mentally is a necessity. It is otherwise impossible to avoid subtle manipulation by mind and emotions in which destiny, God, or other people, are blamed for a responsibility that belongs entirely to the individual.

Process of clarification

If we consider the functioning of the five senses, of which the mind is the interpreter, the awareness that needs to be achieved becomes formidable. All five senses have to be individually investigated to obtain a good balance in their interdependence. The functioning of the mind as an interpreter is mainly through mental images.

The process has to begin at the start:

a) I see—
   the act of seeing—
   what is seen

b) I feel—
   the act of feeling—
   what is felt

c) I hear—
   the act of hearing—
   what is heard

d) I taste—
   the act of tasting—
   what is tasted

e) I smell—
   the act of smelling—
   what is smelled

*Taking
responsibility*

The interplay of forces between body and mind becomes more and more evident as the asanas are practiced and difficulties are encountered. The yoga student gains control in dealing with problems, obstacles, hindrances, and thereby takes full responsibility for progress, timing, achievements, and putting unused faculties into positive action. In other words, a process is set in motion that not only gives a glimpse of human potential, but also puts it within reach.

PERSONALITY ASPECTS

*Cooperating with
one's evolution*

For a long time yoga students may function mainly as their own therapists, with only a little help from a teacher or Guru. A sense of self-worth increases with this active cooperation with one's evolution. The discovery of obstacles by oneself is an important emphasis in Eastern psychology. Its objective is to identify with the Higher Self and thus transcend the many personality aspects that have been imagined as "real entities," impossible to subdue. Dependency and interdependency, of course, do not end here. A variety of spiritual practices is necessary to bring into focus the complexity of Being, particularly being Human.

Identify with the Higher Self

There are many personality aspects in everyone, be it a person with a highly developed intellect, or someone who has been indulging in emotions and ignoring development of the intellect. This process of self-analysis is not for the purpose of judgement, but for a ruthless discovery of the countless personalities and their aspects that are believed to be the real person and, therefore, given authority. The great Masters are emphatic that we are all the creators of our own pain. When we are able to transcend those personality aspects, pain comes to an end.

We create our own pain

Pain can be a great teacher, but only if we are willing to learn. Most of the time our efforts go into avoiding it. In Tadasana, standing still, physical pain is rarely experienced; but emotional pain can be considerable when one just stands and does not know where to go or realizes there is no place to go. Then you may ask yourself, "Have I made enemies, not friends? Have I prided myself on not needing anybody? Were others never my concern? Has selfishness impoverished me?" In the process of clarification these thoughts may confront us painfully.

Pain the teacher

When an undesirable personality aspect has been discovered its power is, by that act, considerably lessened, and transcending it becomes easier. After the decision has been made to deal with the problem, the next phase, applying the will, can be entered. The discriminative faculty of the mind lets one see the difference between self-will (egocentricity) and directed will. Concentration at this point becomes almost effortless. The analytical process clears the field for wider vision, allowing insights to emerge that did not have a chance before because

Will

the "space" was too crowded, the noises of the emotions too loud. The mental-emotional activity volume was too high to hear "the still small voice within."

Reflection not narcissistic

All these thought processes are, of course, centered on the individual, but instead of being narcissistic, they lead to a deeper understanding and control of oneself. "I am the writer of the script of my life." Depressive feelings—like being a leaf the wind blows here and there, crushed by destiny—are bound to lessen, provided the process continues.

REFLECTION

Dreams

The mind's activity, even in sleep, never stops. Dreams show by their contents that the emotions are also ever-present. It would be a good idea to record dreams, especially those that have animals in them, and relate them to the particular asanas that are being practiced. The mental processes that are set in motion by reflection on the meaning of the names of the asanas allow emotional undercurrents to surface and be dealt with in either the waking or sleeping state.

The unconscious throws off ballast

One has only to read the reflections written by members of a yoga class to see the efforts of the unconscious to use this quiet, relaxed time to throw off as much ballast as possible. This opportunity is intentionally created in traditional yogic practice by daily reflection on events, pleasant and unpleasant. The concrete thinker (who sees the cat in the mind) can do so more easily than the abstract thinker (c-a-t).

Symbolic meanings of the asanas

It is during the time of reflection that one can use the symbolic meanings of the postures and their names to deal with irritations and problems, taking time to digest and accept what is, and discovering that one indeed has the power to change things in oneself as well as in life situations. For those who have been very discouraged, a sense of hope grows as they realize that they can DO something about it. To discover strength—never before suspected—in oneself, provides the will to take responsibility (although in small doses at first, and that is all right).

Human beings the world over are goal-oriented. To increase and enhance the goal is very important in Yoga Psychology. Vivekananda, the first swami to come to America (in 1887 for the conference of world religions), pointed out clearly that to be lukewarm is the worst thing to be; "You are neither in the world nor on the Path." To be lukewarm, indecisive, irregular, keeps one in limbo. Each small victory leads to an improvement in attitude that will also reflect in the body. The postures become less difficult because the approach changes from "I will never be able to do this" to "I will try" or "Yes, I can."

Enhance the goal

The will to live, and to make life worthwhile, is a goal that will be brought about by the practice of Yoga. Hatha Yoga, with constant reflection on the asanas themselves and the meaning of the symbolism embedded therein, will bring transcendence of the recognized personality aspects.

Transcending personality aspects

SYMBOLISM IN DAILY LIFE

The emotional impact of symbols may assault concepts already well set in the individual's mind. These concepts may immediately be defended verbally. If intensely felt, the concepts get tucked away in the mind; but they still radiate power and will emerge at a later time.

Symbols assault concepts

Words, which are themselves symbols expressing underlying ideas, are never limited to an assigned meaning. They are the property of everyone and are more often used carelessly than intelligently. Groups may attempt to give words exclusive meanings for specific purposes, but this never limits their influence. Language refuses to be packed into little boxes by the conceptualizations of human beings.

Deeper meanings of words

Symbolic expression does not belong exclusively to the artist, as may be thought. It is important to speculate on the meaning of symbols oneself. In time, that search may also lead one away through fascination with the discovery of endless possibilities that the mind can conjure up for creating, imagining, dreaming, expressing. The mind calls attention to itself by pointing to its capacity to create, making a dazzling display like the sun's many rays.

Symbolizing can be seen as clothing ideas and observations in sometimes precise, sometimes ponderable forms, and as presenting new insights and helping reflections to crystallize.

Power of the mind to change the body

The human body can be influenced, changed, not as an artist does by the stroke of a brush, but by the powers of the mind. A body that is very "dense" will show these influences only faintly, while one that is "loose" can change to an astonishing degree. When given the right attention, the process of change in the body, even to the point of restoring health, will prove this. Where, then, should we put our attention? The following are some suggestions with which you could begin:

How to work with mind and body

1) Study and look at the characteristics of your mind to understand its subtle influences.
2) Scrutinize these influences on the physical body.
3) Observe influences on and by the immediate environment, such as people, living quarters, work, work habits, kinds of entertainment, and relaxation.
4) Find out what all these asanas mean to you.

Working with the shoulderstand

When repeatedly practiced while watching the interaction of the body AND the mind, the shoulderstand will bring many insights:

Salamba Sarvangasana—upside down . . .

upside down, can't move;
upside down, no choice;
upside down, looking—without, within;
upside down, taking stock;
upside down, observing . . .
upside down, feeling . . .
upside down, seeing . . .

upside down, asking: Where am I?
upside down, asking: Where do I want to be?
upside down, asking: Where do I want to go?
upside down, asking: What do I want to do about
myself?

This is only a simple example, yet it will be a start so that one will not become discouraged by the still-apparent complexity. It is also a yogic principle that those practicing Yoga must be encouraged to discover unknown territory by themselves. Even in the most talented, feelings of inferiority are strong. These feelings are not eradicated by rationalizing, but by the actual experience of self-observation. A poor self-image is diminished in the same manner. Positive personal experience through one's own efforts will, under the hammer of repetition, slowly chip away undesirable characteristics. The subtle, negative psychological influences which were so firmly established by repetitive thoughts are now replaced with new building blocks for constructing a different self-image and a feeling of self-worth. Building character and laying a foundation were demanded by the old Masters of all their disciples. Those who listen and indeed follow become masters in their own right.

Self-discovery and self-observation

    The reference material provided with the asanas is given so that each individual can use it to expand and deepen understanding. Write down the thoughts that come to mind and reflect on them later, as they provide valuable insights into oneself.

Using the reference notes

    However, a decision of will has to be made to put all this valuable fact-finding into action to bring about the intended change. The desire for this change has to be given the now-positive power of the emotions, and must be continuously nourished by daily action, observations, and clarification.

Act on insights

    What is called "the Path" today is just this ongoing process. There is simply NO magical formula that will bring results without effort. With practice, the individual matures and learns to accept facts, however disconcerting they may be. One

Results require effort

Trim needs

of the most distressing discoveries by yoga students is that needs have to be trimmed like fruit trees, lest they become g-r-e-e-d. The discriminatory faculties have to be applied in order for one to become very clear about this aspect.

*Taking
responsibility for
oneself*

It is necessary to remember that while life-styles change (as when a society becomes industrialized), human beings change with the tide of those times only according to their sense of inner worth. Those who cannot make an adjustment are the casualties. These changes have forced people to take responsibility for themselves in a more holistic way. Many have turned to other cultures to learn what could be gained from them, to find a different perspective.

*Essence of Hatha
Yoga*

The interplay of forces between the body and the mind is undeniable, even if imperceptible for a long time. We cannot see our physical body grow, and yet it DOES grow. There is also no doubt that bodily activities do influence the mind. Running, swimming, or dancing give a lift, while chanting, singing, or laughing bring about a more subtle influence. When an asana is mastered, intelligence serves a new purpose as awareness streams with its help into every fiber, every cell of the body. There is a new sense of being united with one's body and self. The essence of Hatha Yoga is achieved.

1. Indian culture is too complex a topic to be dealt with here. Consult the Bibliography for sources.

2. The Kundalini system refers to an ancient and precise discipline that can lead to Higher Consciousness. It uses a symbolic language to describe levels of consciousness (chakras). The chakras will be mentioned from time to time in this book. For more on the Kundalini system see Swami Sivananda Radha, *Kundalini: Yoga for the West*.

3. See Sivananda Radha, *Mantras: Words of Power*.

4. See the second last paragraph of *A Word from the Author*.

5. The hidden influences in the postures exert a kind of subtle pressure (massage) which, it has been discovered, is similar in acupuncture.

6. Kuvalayananda, *Yoga Therapy*, 24.

7. Iyengar, *Light on Yoga*, 22.

8. Patanjali's system of Raja Yoga identifies eight limbs of Yoga which, if practiced, will allow an aspirant to develop into a well-balanced being. The eight limbs involve physical, ethical, and mental practices. See the Bibliography for books written by Wood, Vivekananda, and Taimni on Raja Yoga.

9. Maslow, "A Philosophy of Psychology."

10. For more on this, see Walsh and Vaughan, *Beyond Ego: Transpersonal Dimensions in Psychology*.

11. Green, "On the Meaning of Transpersonal," 37.

12. Balkin, "Belief and the Management of Chronic Pain," 41.

13. See Sivananda Radha, *Kundalini: Yoga for the West*.

14. Mindwatching: This can be done for ten minutes by closing the eyes and watching what happens before the "mental eye." The next ten minutes are then used to write down what the watcher has observed. Depending on the result, it may be necessary to repeat this exercise many times to get a good understanding of the working of one's mind. The written material will also reveal hindrances that are likely to be serious problems that have to be dealt with before concentration can be achieved. These problems will most likely express themselves in the body: fear of doing an exercise, inability to bend in a particular way or turn in a given direction, etc.

YOGA PSYCHOLOGY

STRUCTURES

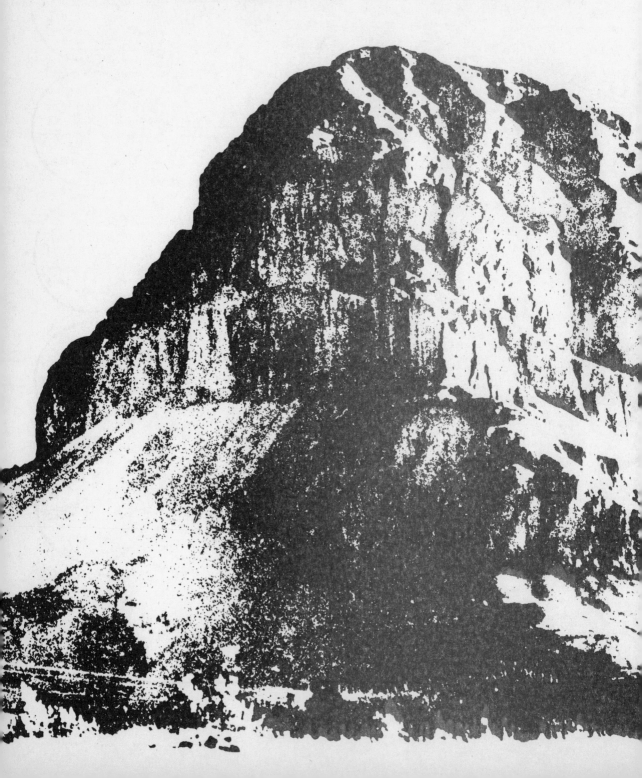

tadasana

MOUNTAIN

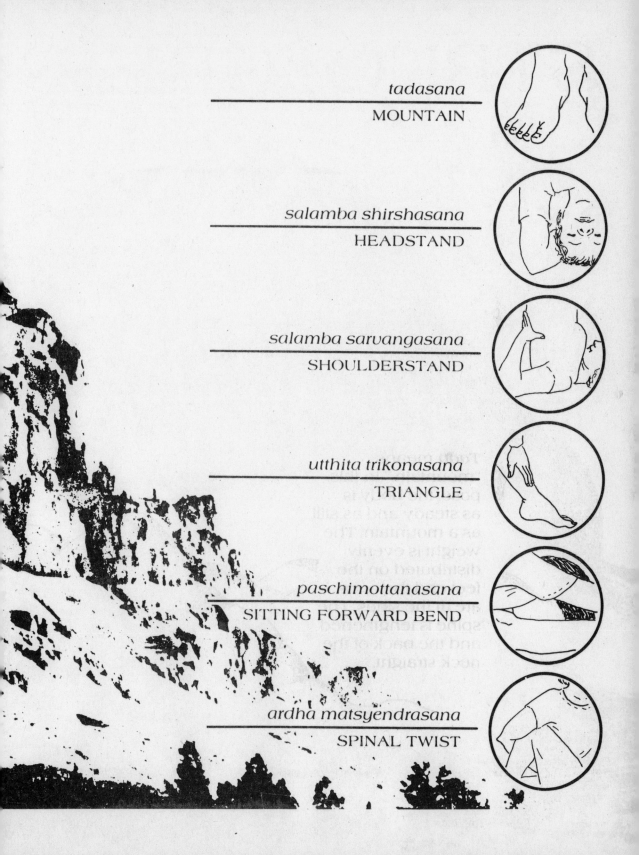

salamba shirshasana

HEADSTAND

salamba sarvangasana

SHOULDERSTAND

utthita trikonasana

TRIANGLE

paschimottanasana

SITTING FORWARD BEND

ardha matsyendrasana

SPINAL TWIST

Tada means "mountain." In this pose, the body is as steady and as still as a mountain. The weight is evenly distributed on the feet and the arms are at the sides. The spine is lengthened and the back of the neck straight.

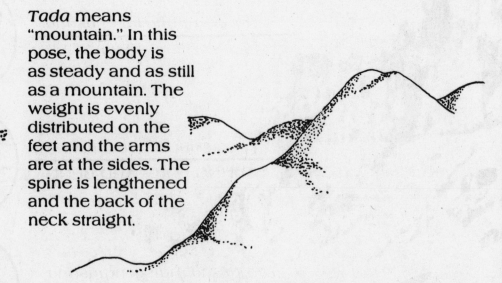

tadasana

MOUNTAIN

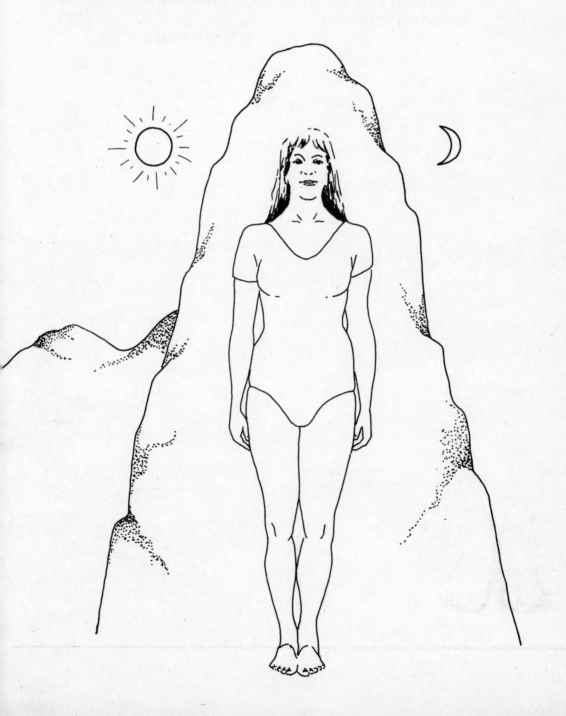

"Nobody can go to heaven unless the foundation is firm."

B.K.S. Iyengar

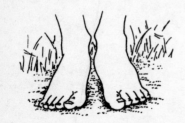

tadasana

MOUNTAIN

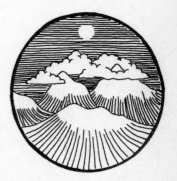

IN PRACTICING AN ASANA the focus may be simultaneously on the sense of feeling, the body, the mind, and what is termed "myself." In Tadasana, attention can first be given to the meaning of the name: MOUNTAIN, STANDING UP, STANDING STILL. It will become quite evident that the mind is not willing, able, or in the mood to CONCENTRATE. Several phases are involved. The mind is like a central station where everything pours in that the senses perceive, and it has to make interpretations from those perceptions. There are many choices for the mind to make. In this case it must find the meaning for the aspirant of *mountain* and *standing still.* Here is an example of how to do this:

TADASANA: Mountain Posture
*Standing still, upright—awareness of body,
muscles, ligaments, bones, structure, being erect,
different from animal, holding together,
balancing, resting, pull, push, stomach, swaying,
compulsion to move, arrested movement,
stillness*

These are good simple starters to help the individual to think in areas that may have been neglected for too long.

The first thought is, I am standing . . . here . . . still. . . . Only after this acknowledgement can the idea of mountain occur, and "what a mountain means to me."

Tadasana—standing still, when repeatedly practiced with observations on the body AND the mind, will bring many insights:

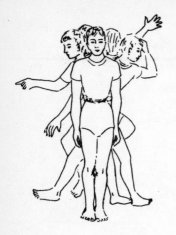

standing still, not running somewhere;
standing still, looking—without, within;
standing still, taking stock;
standing still, observing . . .
standing still, feeling . . .
standing still, seeing . . .
standing still, asking: Where am I?
standing still, asking: Where do I want to be?
standing still, asking: Where do I want to go?
standing still, asking: What do I want to do about
myself?

For some people words may tumble into the mind: immensity, power, great strength, obstacles, avalanches, destruction. For others the words come slowly, like beads on a string, with only a vague meaning attached to them. Depending on the strength of the accompanying emotions, those ideas/words are pursued further, or fade. Personal associations may surface, such as: being alone, lost in the mountains, there is nobody there to "stand" by. It is not unusual for a person to be suddenly overcome by this kind of thought, because in general people keep themselves busy in order to avoid thinking too much.

When the mountain is a symbol for obstacles, preventing vision or perspective, emotions like fear can run very deep. The obstacles in life may appear "mountainous" with no one standing by. When one begins thinking about oneself with the help of symbols, awareness comes little by little; or in the case of "I am alone," with the overpowering strength of a mountain. We are, of course, always alone; we are born alone and die alone. If this thought is disconcerting, it is because it has been suppressed from awareness. Reflections of this kind are a good preparation for meditation. In fact, for most people, meditation is more like reflection.

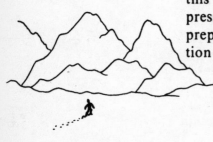

tadasana

MOUNTAIN

TADASANA: Mountain Posture

*Standing up, standing straight, looking ahead,
facing what is in front, keeping balanced,
resisting movement, running away from,
becoming aware of the body that stands erect,
raised from a slumped position, depression,
shoulders stooped from carrying weight—whose
weight? wanting to stretch beyond what limits?*

What is a mountain made of? Heaps of earth, rock, compressed stuff of an enormous size. A mountain is immovable, a frightening rise, apparently haphazardly structured, invoking the image of possible avalanches under which one could be buried. Are these like my insurmountable problems which have been allowed to accumulate and compress? Descending the mountain, giving up, looking down at the terrifying steepness; ascending the mountain, finding a way, growing, the exhilaration of the view from the elevation . . . contrasting pictures in the mind. Up or down, good or bad, disaster or success, all these thoughts lead to moderating the mind as well as the emotions.

TADASANA: Mountain Posture

*Space to stand on, space above, space all around;
who stands—a person? an actor? a shell?
a ghost? where do I stand? standing up for
myself, for someone else; being true,
straightforward; where do I stand on important
principles, ideals, ethics, decisions, beliefs,
convictions? do I stand on my own two feet?*

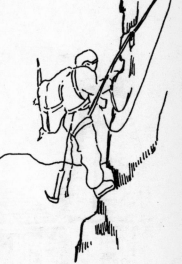

The mountaineer is challenged by the awesomeness of the mountain, and by the obstacles that it presents—taking pride in achieving, in the idea of conquering the mountain—until fear is conquered by accepting the challenge and surmounting the difficulties.

REFLECTIONS: Mountain Aspiration

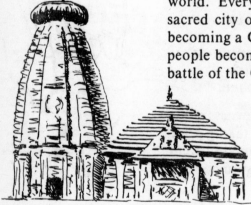

Who is not inspired by the view of a snow-capped mountain? Mountains have greatness and dignity. To ascend a mountain demands an optimum of strength and stamina. Mount Everest with its tremendous physical challenge lures many mountaineers. Nearby is a legendary holy mountain, Annapurna, which presents the same kind of challenge for the spiritual aspirant.

The mountain is a symbol of the aspiration to transcend one's little self. It also stands for purity and selflessness. The process of ascent is a spiritual pursuit toward a solitude in which the rational mind must surrender its dominance. All intellectual activity has to recede to allow the mind periodically to be in its original state. Here at an elevated place is found quiet for meditation, for going within—rising above the dualism that invites constant battles between the head and the heart.[1] And yet that dualism is psychologically necessary to gain knowledge through certain experiences that are above positive and negative.

The mountain is a symbol for more than transcendental imagery. As the symbol of the Center, "The Sacred Mountain —where heaven and earth meet—is situated at the center of the world. Every temple or palace—and, by extension, every sacred city or royal residence—is a Sacred Mountain, thus becoming a Center."[2] Ashrams and their residences for holy people become the center, the meeting ground, on which the battle of the Gita is fought.

tadasana

MOUNTAIN

With its valleys, ledges, and numerous caves, the remnants of underground streams, the mountain tells the story of how, for thousands of years, it has benefited all who have lived on it. The caves have given shelter to seekers who have retreated into them to enter the solitude that allows communion between those two worlds—that of the individual and of the surrounding world—to listen to the rocks sing, the rumble of the mountain spirit, or the voice of the prophets.[3]

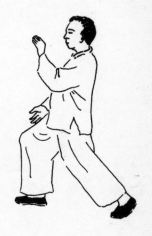

In the caves of the mountain occurs the transformation that takes one beyond the rational mind. This is a process of rebirth. It is like retiring into an enormous womb, to emerge anew.[4] For those who would go to the mountains to spend time in seclusion for meditation, who have the stamina and courage to retreat in this way, the ascent can be the preparation. Whatever one's accomplishment in Hatha Yoga, Tadasana—the mountain posture—can lead one through the maze of thoughts and remove the obstacles, to achieve the first rung of the ladder. Like Tadasana, the T'ai Chi posture "Return to Mountain" symbolizes a return to the inner stillness that gives one the power to climb beyond the ego.

The mountain, then, symbolizes the ascent toward the goal one wants to attain. Mountains, as the abode of the gods, are comparable to the sources of wisdom from which knowledge radiates in all directions, like rivers that flow from the mountain to fertilize the land.

The gods who supposedly reside on the mountains may at one time have been human beings who rose above mediocrity to realize a potential they recognized within themselves.[5] These gods, geniuses in spiritual evolution, provide the balance of quietude for the restlessness of the world and its mental-emotional activity. Within this polarity, each complements the other. In *The I Ching,* the fifty-second hexagram is called "Kên/Keeping Still, Mountain." In its application to man, the hexagram turns upon the problem of achieving a quiet heart.

tadasana

MOUNTAIN

Quietness will surface and, by this new process of thinking, the mind will recede a little at a time. One has to be ever on the alert not to be caught in an avalanche or mountain slide, under which everything is buried. Confidence must not become over-confidence and, while risks have to be taken, they must not be reckless, but tempered with the power of discrimination, with the strong desire for clear vision. Then one will be like the Greek gods on Mount Olympus.

Mount Meru represents, for the Hindus, the axis around which the world turns, motionlessness within constant motion, the impenetrable paradoxes. Kailasa[6] is the abode of Shiva, Lord of Yoga, called the great Compassionate Lord. Devoted Hindus wish to make a pilgrimage to Kailasa once in their lifetime. It was at Mount Kailasa that Vivekananda had a vision of Lord Shiva, which he could not transmit to his disciple, Sister Nivedita, who accompanied him on that pilgrimage. Vivekananda cried out in agony at the recognition that he did not have the power of his great Master, Ramakrishna, who was able to transmit knowledge.

A mountain like Vesuvius can be alive with an inner fire. Where passion for the Most High burns within the aspirant like a volcano, an inner explosion throws out the ashes of things that are no longer needed.

Swedenborg, the modern mystic (1772), says that mountains are to be understood "in the good of love, by reason that the angels dwell upon mountains; such as are in love to the Lord dwelling on high mountains, and such as are in love to their neighbor dwelling on lower ones; wherefore by every mountain is signified every good of love."[7]

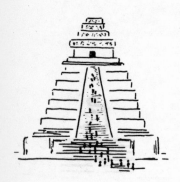

People of the deserts and plains where there are no mountains, as in Egypt, the Yucatan, and South America, have attempted elevation by building pyramids—structured mountains. On top of the mountain or pyramid there is a wider vision. Everything diminishes to its proper size and loses its exaggerated importance. The mountain never moves; it seems to stand there solidly forever. Yet mountains do move, imperceptibly—except for avalanches or eruptions. The division between the movable and the immovable vanishes. Elevating thoughts appear from the horizon as from nowhere and these take one to the mountaintop within.

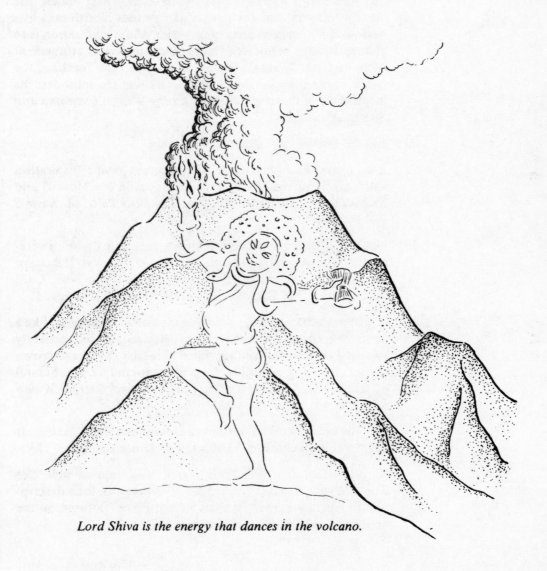

Lord Shiva is the energy that dances in the volcano.

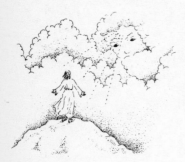

1. "In this epoch, perhaps more than in any past epoch, the city-dwelling multitudes need that spiritual rebirth which is bestowed by Earth's sacred mountains. If our civilization is to endure, it must break its urban fetters and live in attunement with the Great Mother. It must know as do the Teachers, the music of the silences, the companionship of the solitudes, the inspiration of the High Places." Evans-Wentz, *Cuchama and Sacred Mountains,* 33.

2. Eliade, *Cosmos and History,* 12.

3. Two examples of prophets who received divine inspiration while on a mountain are Jesus (Sermon on the Mount) and Moses (Ten Commandments). See *The Holy Bible,* Matthew 5 and Exodus 19.

4. The Himalayas symbolize the female aspect of Creation's tremendous power through Mena, the wife of Himavat (Himalaya personified), and Parvati, their daughter, who won Lord Shiva's heart. See Dimmitt, *Classical Hindu Mythology,* 157.

5. "Each of the mountains encircling the Earth is placed . . . like a never sleeping and silent tutelary deity eagerly but patiently awaiting that far-distant age when mankind shall have grown to the full stature of godhood, here in mankind's divine School of the World." Evans-Wentz, *Cuchama and Sacred Mountains,* 11.

6. " . . . the most sacred mountain to Hindus and Buddhists. . . . It has never been climbed." Tobias, *The Mountain Spirit,* 213.

Native Americans have their sacred mountain as well. See Evans-Wentz, *Cuchama and Sacred Mountains,* for a description of Cuchama, the "Exalted Sacred Place," located on the border between California and Mexico.

For an inspiring description of the sacred mountain, see Lama Anagarika Govinda's *The Way of the White Clouds*. The following is a brief excerpt from part 5, chapter 1, "The Sacred Mountain":

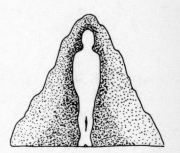

> Personality consists in the power to influence others, and this power is due to consistency, harmony, and one-pointedness of character. If these qualities are present in a mountain we recognise it as a vessel of cosmic power, and we call it a sacred mountain.
>
> The power of such a mountain is so great and yet so subtle that, without compulsion, people are drawn to it from near and far, as if by the force of some invisible magnet; and they will undergo untold hardships and privations in their inexplicable urge to approach and to worship the centre of this sacred power. . . .
>
> Instead of conquering it the religious-minded man prefers to be conquered by the mountain. He opens his soul to its spirit and allows it to take possession of him. . . .
>
> There are some [mountains] of such outstanding character and position that they become symbols of the highest aspirations of humanity, as expressed in ancient civilisations and religions, milestones of the eternal quest for perfection and ultimate realisation.

7.   Gaskell, *Dictionary of All Scriptures and Myths*, 516.

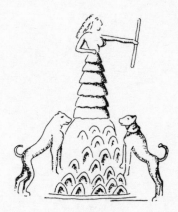

Cybele, Great Mother of Asia Minor and Goddess of the World Mountain

Salamba means "with support." *Shirsha* means "head." In this pose, the forearms are on the floor, the hands clasped and cupped to form a place for the head to rest. The legs are raised perpendicular to the floor, the spine is lengthened, and the weight evenly distributed on the arms and head.

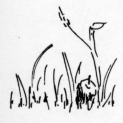

salamba shirshasana

HEADSTAND

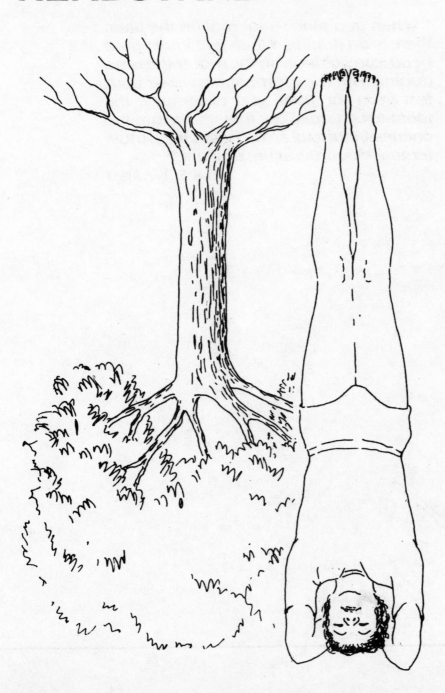

"When you place your mat on the floor, there is no duality. When you lower your head into position on the mat, there is no duality. But the moment you raise your feet from the floor, you experience the identity of 'I'; take out that and retain the oneness, that total awareness which must remain throughout the posture."

B.K.S. Iyengar

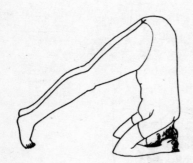

salamba shirshasana

HEADSTAND

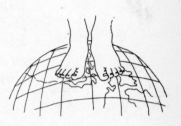

Y<small>OUR FEET ARE</small> the foundation on which you stand. As an earth-dweller, standing on the earth, that is where you have your roots, as well as in a particular country, city, or place. What does it mean to be earth-bound? You are subject to the needs of the body, to gravitational influences, and to the numerous interferences the earth exercises—climate, sunshine, rain, wind, day, night.

We have evolved from the animal kingdom, which is subject to the same influences. But the yogi says there must be more. The human brain has been carefully prepared to enable the human being to become the receptacle of the Divine Spark. From that spark, the inception before conception, slowly comes the beginning of awareness, the process of growth and development—your own individual process of learning.

The seat of that spark, the jiva, is in the brain; the skull contains the brain. The head is connected with the feet through the body and its various systems. To develop that jiva, one has to uproot oneself by turning the concepts of life and purpose of living upside down. In the headstand, that which has been rooted in the earth becomes rooted in heaven. The nourishment that came from the earth is now supplied by greater forces from above.

In this posture, familiar surroundings are seen upside down. This may cause some unpleasantness, different emotions—even fear. Rebellion may emerge powerfully in a struggle to defend views and cherished beliefs. Everything is at the opposite end from what used to be the best and only "right" way. Comfort and security are challenged. This is difficult to accept.

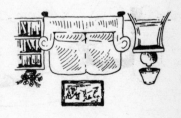

You may find yourself thinking, What would happen if my life were turned upside down? I am standing on my head—how do my strong convictions look now? In this position like an upside down tree, I can't move. Do I know where I am rooted?

SALAMBA SHIRSHASANA: Headstand Posture

Upside down, struggle, rebellion, defences, fear,
Divine Spark, awareness, process of growth,
learning; brain, head, body, feet—connections;
rooted in earth; rooted in heaven? uprooted

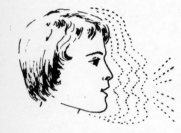

Standing on the head brings clarity of mind, not only in regard to emotions, but also speech. Powerful suggestions by word or thought will surface and show their often-devastating influence, sometimes bordering on a kind of self-hypnosis. Like the blood as it rushes to the brain bringing large amounts of oxygen, this realization can wipe clean the grooves of habitual thinking.

When you have your head on the ground, you cannot live in the clouds. Whatever you do, whatever you discover, must be well-grounded and stand the test of examination. The tools for that examination are reason and logic, and their use contributes to the process of learning.

When your feet, which were symbolically rooted in the earth, become rooted in heaven, the nourishment you receive is no longer intellectual or even philosophical, but spiritual. To be rooted in heaven means to receive nourishment from the Divine. It means to be rooted in the ideals and ethics that you have established for yourself.

As you learn balance and courage in the practice of the posture, realize that the pressure you feel in the asana is your own body, and that the burdens in life are your own; it is not your task to carry the weight of, or the responsibility for, anyone else. What are your burdens? What is the psychological implication of looking at them from a different perspective?

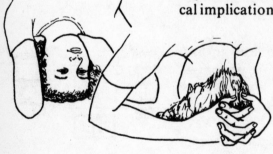

After doing the exercise, having looked at your familiar surroundings upside down, write your reactions—how you feel and what you think. If in this process you meet with strong opposition to your convictions, become your own opponent, take the other side of the argument. Having done so, there will be no need to argue with others. By being your own opponent you will have already recognized a powerful emotional attachment. It would be good to write down your insights and how you are going to act on them. In this reverse position, facing fears before they can materialize means finding options. It is precisely those attachments and cherished beliefs that keep one intentionally blind to the fact that there are often many options in a difficult or dramatic situation.

SALAMBA SHIRSHASANA: Headstand Posture

Rooted in heaven, space for my roots; learning balance and courage; is my head in the clouds? well-grounded, reason, logic; emotional reactions, cherished beliefs, intentional blindness; what are my burdens? are they really mine?

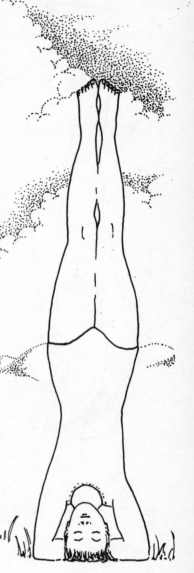

The physical benefits of this asana also soon become obvious. The body gains in strength, flexibility, and grace of movement; the complexion improves; you become generally healthier. Because of the inverted posture, the blood rushes to the head, nourishing the brain, supplying extra oxygen. The teeth, gums, and all the organs located in the head are also benefited and strengthened. From a yogic point of view, however, these are not the most important reasons for doing the headstand.

Having your head on the ground, well-rooted, means having an intellect that is well-developed and practical. When your feet are rooted in heaven instead of the earth, inspiration will stand the test of practical application, and increased intuitive perception will help you to meet new complex situations.

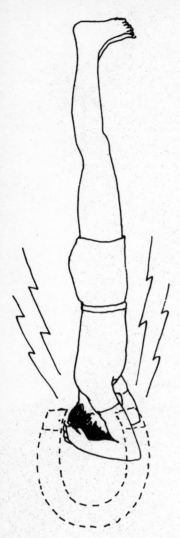

Increased awareness makes it quite clear that great inspirations do not come from the ego, which is in fact the source of all problems and difficulties. There is more flexibility when you are rooted in your new ways of thinking; it cannot be helped that in the beginning you will substitute one set of convictions for another, until greater awareness has led you to the Light within.

It takes a long time before freedom and independence are easily accepted and one feels comfortable with them. These words, *freedom* and *liberation,* must be clarified by each individual. The key to freedom of any kind is in our own hands. Yoga in its many forms offers such a key, and the various practices help one to accept the responsibility for that freedom.

Once you have learned to do this posture in a relaxed manner, you will gain an understanding of balance in your life and of the union of two worlds: the world of the body and that of the mind. The insights that come to you in Hatha Yoga will gradually go beyond the purely physical. The mind and the center of consciousness have to become a magnet to attract the great Light of Consciousness, so that the body will become a spiritual tool and you will receive the nectar and ambrosia of divine inspiration.

REFLECTIONS: Headstand

It is necessary to grasp the psychological aspects of the headstand in order to understand the mystical or spiritual aspects. You may think, when you stand with your feet securely placed on the earth, that you stand firmly to meet the demands of daily life. But this concept must be reversed in the headstand.

Before doing the posture, invoke in your mind's eye the image of a tree turned upside down—the roots are in the air and the crown on the earth.[1] Think of the trunk of the tree as your spine. Your head, which is on the ground, is the thousand-petalled lotus and contains the brain where all sense input is interpreted. The base of your spine is the seat of energy, the first chakra,[2] the source of nectar and ambrosia. When this nectar and ambrosia reaches the head, divine insights and inspiration occur. In the third lotus, or chakra, located in the solar plexus, the energy used by the emotions is like a flame; but in this position the aspirant cannot feed this flame to keep it burning. There are many movements (to fulfill ambitions and gratify desires) that cannot be made since you are almost immovable when standing on your head. In the normal upright position the mind sees the attraction of the world through the senses and the Light cannot enter. Divine inspirations fall into the fire of passion and are burned. In the headstand they are preserved, and the nectar and ambrosia are not lost in that fire; the divine energy can be properly used.

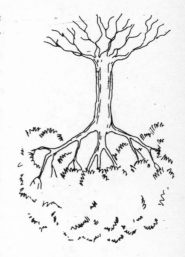

When you stand on your head think, This is a different form of surrender. And, for the first three chakras particularly: I surrender all the entertainment, excitement, and what I consider to be great fun. I will investigate these things. I will find out how much importance I have given to each through the power of illusion, through the power of desire. How do I create desires? How do I feed desires?

The Devi of Speech[3] becomes an important part of this investigation. Is my desire for expression just giving in to the demands of the ego? Through the practice of asanas one eliminates the verbal chatter and sees its needlessness. The desire grows to reverse as much as possible all sense stimulation. The headstand is excellent for this. All the movements to get into the posture have a significance. Bending over from a standing position to place the head, the seat of the intellect, on the ground, is symbolic for humility. It is almost like doing

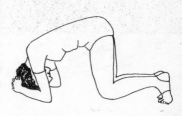

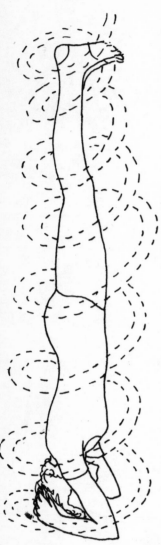

obeisance to the Divine. The feet and legs, the foundation, are lifted off the ground until they are vertical. Raising the feet in the air is surrendering the security of the earth. For this period of time one cannot take off into flights of fancy, nor respond to the stimulation of the senses. It is such an unaccustomed posture, removing oneself from one's firm foundation, that it demands full attention to maintain. The balance required is very difficult. As in other asanas, limitations are obvious as one becomes aware of muscles, joints, and bones in a different way.

Moderation and quality of life form the first gateway through which one enters to receive the nectar and ambrosia. That still small voice within, the spiritual insights, come in moments of quietness when there is no activity of the mind, when the merry-go-round has been stopped. When you take a normal position once more, having explored the reverse position fully, you will have discovered that basic nourishment comes from higher sources, whether it is called God, the Absolute, Cosmic Intelligence, or your Divine Committee.

A powerful mystical aspect of the headstand is the movement of pranic energy in the body.[4] When the position can be held easily, it should be connected with some spiritual thought. An Eastern Mantra may be used, or the aspirant may choose something from his or her religious background. This becomes a kind of energy which moves around in the whole body, a tiny pinpoint of Light invigorating the body and giving it extra vitality.

Awareness of this energy in your daily life counteracts the psychological effect of being rooted in the earth, so that every moment becomes miraculous. You will be able to see the miracle of your hand—all the things that you can do with it; that beautiful apparatus that you call your eye; or the magic mirror of your mind—your imagination. The human body is then seen as a marvelous tool, to be respected and cared for, not taken for granted.

1. The image of an inverted tree found in the *Bhagavad Gita* (15:1-2) and the *Katha Upanishad* (6:1) is not unique to the Indian mind. Joseph Campbell in *The Mythic Image* (192) has found Middle Eastern and Western parallels in the *Kabbalah* and in the writings of John of Ruysbroeck and Dante.

   "The idea of an erect and of an inverted tree is met with over a range of time and space extending from Plato to Dante and Siberia to India and Melanesia." *Coomaraswamy. I: Selected Papers*, 386.

2. See Swami Sivananda Radha, *Kundalini: Yoga for the West*, for an explanation of the chakras.

3. Ibid.

4. "Prana [is] life force, often interpreted as breath. Prana is consciousness, the most subtle life-essence that pervades all manifested forms. Prana is the sum total of all existing energy in the universe, that primal Energy manifest, unmanifest, or in a nuclear state." Ibid., 211.

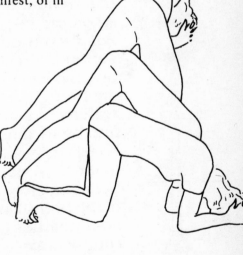

salamba shirshasana

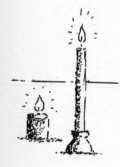

Sarva means "whole, entire."
Anga means "limb" or "body."
Salamba means "with a prop or
support." From a relaxed lying
down position, the legs and torso
are brought to a vertical position
with the weight on the shoulders
and head. If necessary, the
hands may support the back.
In the final stage, the arms are
held vertically by the sides
of the body. The shoulderstand
is sometimes called the
candle pose.

salamba sarvangasana
SHOULDERSTAND

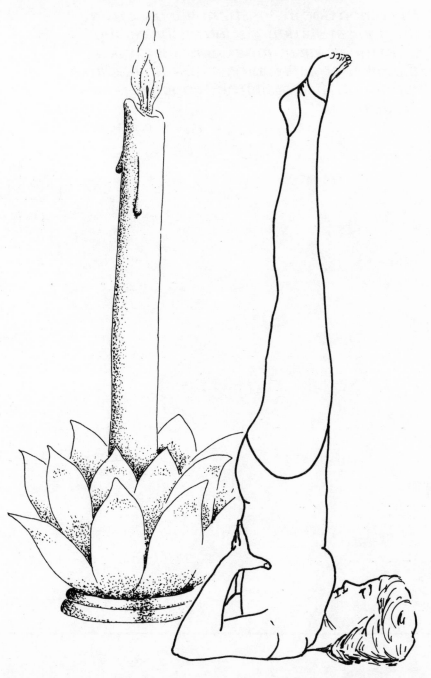

"Position God in Paschimottanasana on the floor, in Sarvangasana on the ceiling. . . . In the same manner, you can think of the inflow or outflow of breath in Kumbhaka as though His Totality had engulfed your entire body."

B.K.S. Iyengar

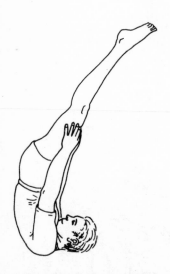

salamba sarvangasana

SHOULDERSTAND

THE SHOULDERSTAND, unlike Tadasana, is an inverted posture. There takes place in the body a reversal of its functioning, with the mind being drawn into it because, as in the headstand, there is no choice. Being upside down also demands a greater sense of balance, a different kind of control of the muscles, and strength in the spine.

It is not the width or the strength of the shoulders themselves that allows one to do the shoulderstand well; it is rather the flexibility of the neck and throat. This flexibility permits the head to remain flat on the floor while the body is perpendicular. The throat is the seat of self-will. This asana is very difficult for many because it involves the bending of the will.

The pressure of the body in the shoulderstand makes the veins in the head swell. The discomfort forces the mind to focus. And the security that we just thought we had found, sitting or standing, is once again shaken when the feet and legs are taken off the ground and the bend is shifted from the lower body to the shoulders.

SALAMBA SARVANGASANA:
Shoulderstand Posture

Inverted, reversal, no choice, upside down, balance, control, strength, shoulder width, bending the will, flexibility, pressure, discomfort, security; feeling shaken, didn't know I was so stiff-necked, trying to hold my legs steady, think I'm going to suffocate

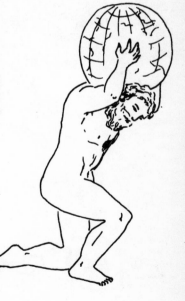

When we think of shoulders, we think first of our own, and how much in life we have to shoulder—responsibility, pain, and loss. We may become aware that self-importance often causes us to shoulder responsibilities that are not ours.

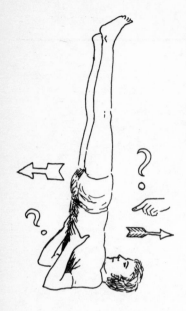

But it also becomes evident that the shoulders and the neck are able to carry the burdens they need to carry.

The back of the head being pushed against the ground is rather like being up against a wall. There is compression on the neck and head; and the gravitational influences that are always present become more noticeable. This reversal of the weight and its pressures may bring to attention the wrong choices that have been made in life.

Standing in an unusual position such as the shoulderstand is like a warning to be prepared for the unusual or extraordinary that happens in other moments of life. The tool of discrimination becomes important once again.

SALAMBA SARVANGASANA: Shoulderstand Posture

Responsibility, pain, and loss; self-importance, against a wall, wrong choices, compression, gravitational influences, burdens, warning, extraordinary, discrimination, movement, change, walking lighter, lending a shoulder, shoulder-width apart

One cannot stand forever on the shoulders. Remember as you move back into another position that life is movement, that nothing lasts forever, and that there is always something changing in the body as well as in the mind. As you come down from Salamba Sarvangasana, let your focus be, What burdens can I put down? What burdens are no longer mine?—so that you may walk lighter on the path of self-development.

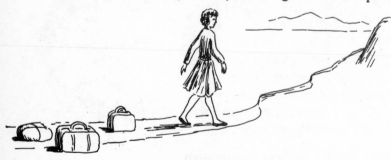

Dramatic moments of life may bring us the opportunity willingly to take on the burden of someone in need, lending them our shoulder as a support in time of trouble. While thinking about the meaning of this asana, we can see the need not only for our own independence, but also for our interdependence through interaction with others. It is then we realize that we are indeed only shoulder-width apart.

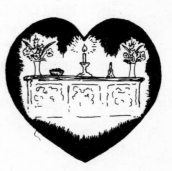

REFLECTIONS: Shoulderstand

When everything is comfortable and pleasant human beings become complacent. It is being under pressure that makes us sit up and think of what has yet to be done to reach our goal. Awareness is not increased one iota unless we are put under pressure.

Pains in the neck are either self-created or come from others who will not bend to our will. The surrender that we must make to the asana is a symbol for the surrender of our self-will to the Most High. As the physical pressure is released, the body comes into balance; similarly, as the ego lets go of the weight that, in its self-importance, it has imagined, the burden is removed. As convictions and strong opinions allow themselves to be swayed, we realize that there is no up, there is no down. The authority of the self-will is undermined.

Sometimes this pose has been called the *candle pose*. That summarizes it very beautifully: I can help to "lighten" myself. Let the spiritual flame, then, burn day and night in the tabernacle of my heart, the meeting place of the two worlds in which I must live. And let my self-will be the first offering to be brought to the altar of life itself, so that, as the first step, consideration of others will lead me to acceptance and love.

Utthita means "extended," *tri* means "three," and *kona* is "an angle." This is the extended triangle, which is done first to one side and then to the other. The legs spread apart and the body stretches to the left, moving from the pelvis and extending over the left leg. Both arms are perpendicular to the floor, the left hand on the floor, or grasping the outer ankle of the left foot, and the right hand reaching up straight. The spine is straight, the chest is open, the body facing to the front.

utthita trikonasana
TRIANGLE

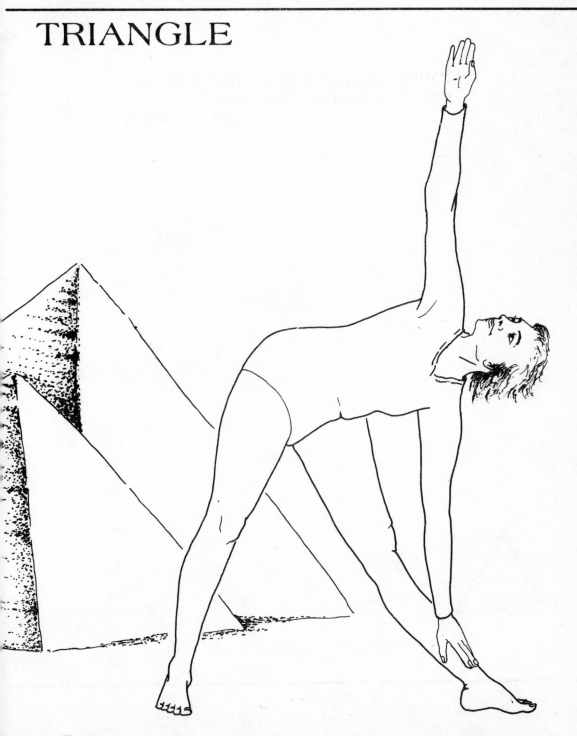

"*Mind, spirit and body have to be one: three in one, and one in three.*"

B.K.S. Iyengar

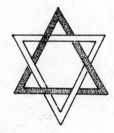

utthita trikonasana

TRIANGLE

IT IS FASCINATING to see again, through the practice of this asana, how the body and the world around it are interconnected. The triangle posture emphasizes the three parts of the interplay of forces: dependency, interdependency, and interaction.[1]

The triangle appears in many forms in the world. Logicians see language in a triadic relationship—there is a speaker, the thing said, and the one spoken to. In religion, the Godhead as three-in-one is called a *triune*. There might be a connection here to the early Roman government in which a group of three people, either of exceptional capacities or of world fame, formed a triumvirate. The sea-god, Neptune, has a trident as a symbol of his power, and the ancient Romans used a three-pronged spear in combat. Many islanders also caught fish with such spears.

The qualities of a triangle are strength, and the ability to support weight and resist pressure; and so the principle of the triangle is used extensively in the building industry. As you stand in Utthita Trikonasana, you might ask yourself how much you can support, and how well you can resist pressure.

UTTHITA TRIKONASANA: Triangle Posture

Dependency, interdependency, interaction, three-in-one, trident, power, supremacy, will, sturdy, supportive, resisting pressure, shaky, tense, unsafe, collapsing, anxious

The tripod, used by photographers to steady the camera in order to get sharp pictures, is triangular in structure. When physical balance has been achieved in the practice of this asana, a sharper picture will emerge of the balance required in all areas of life. Originally, a tripod was a caldron with three legs, used for cooking food over a fire. The aspirant needs to be nourished in three areas: body, mind, and spirit. Food is a rather important issue with most people, and usually the body is well fed. The emotions also take their food at every opportunity, and often people feed on each other's emotions. The food for the mind usually comes through the intellect, but that part of the mind in which the contact is made with the God within, commonly termed *spirit,* rarely gets any wholesome food. Spiritual food can be derived from meditation, prayer, and reflection on God in any form: the Christian Trinity—Father, Son, and Holy Spirit—or the Hindu Trinity—Brahma, Shiva, and Vishnu.

UTTHITA TRIKONASANA: Triangle Posture

Tripod, steady, balance, poise, correct focus, sharp pictures, angles, caldron, wholesome food, nourishment—body, mind, spirit; feeding on emotions, reflection, meditation, prayer, trinity

In daily human relationships there is the trinity of father, mother, and child. In times past when infant survival was rare due to primitive conditions, the birth of live triplets was taken as a special blessing of the deity.

The three wheels of a tricycle help the rider in sustaining balance. But in doing the asana, the height, length, and width of the body, legs, and arms are the deciding factors. The harmonious execution of Utthita Trikonasana means that one is well-balanced and properly focused.[2]

REFLECTIONS: Triangle

Triumphal arches—symbols of power, monumental structures having three arches—were erected to commemorate victories. But the victories celebrated the conquering of others instead of conquering oneself. Hatha Yoga, Bhakti Yoga, and Jnana Yoga first appear as separate when they are in fact a single monumental structure that needs to be built into one's life.

If a triangle is placed within a circle, all vertices are touched. Body, mind, and speech are the three vertices which, in the attempt to achieve all-round development, will eventually bring those straight lines into balance. The aspirant will then be within the circle of perfection.

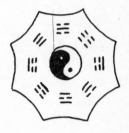

Three lines in different arrangements are called *trigrams* and are used in Chinese and Japanese divination. Although the oracles of the well-known *I Ching* are helpful, they cannot replace the need for going deeply within and touching one's inner source. Three days of prayer, a triduum, sometimes precede spiritual occasions or practices in many religions, and include a fast or special celebrations to prepare oneself for the inner path.

Jesus reminded his followers that where two or three are gathered together, there he would be also. He also told Peter, with sadness, "Thrice you will deny me." This warning appears in other religions as well. The aspirant must heed this warning in order to achieve the promised balance of the asana, to unite in compassion with others, and to achieve the state of the spiritual union (marriage) within.

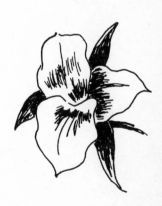

To grow and nourish the trillium, the trinity lily, with its three large white petals, is to nourish the symbol of a pure heart, pure body, and pure mind. Taking the three steps leading up to the tabernacle of the heart will allow love and compassion to flower.

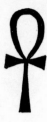

The loop of the ankh, the Egyptian cross, is the symbol of the Life Force, of prana, and of the power of awareness. Let the body dance to the musical trio, the three divine instruments: the vina, the flute, and the drum—the sacred music that counterbalances the chatter of competition. Shiva, the Lord of Yoga, holding the three-pronged scepter, represents the state of Satchitananda (truth, consciousness, bliss) to those who worship him. But what is worship? It is dedication of the body as a spiritual tool, and of the mind as the bridge to another world, to Liberation—Satchitananda.

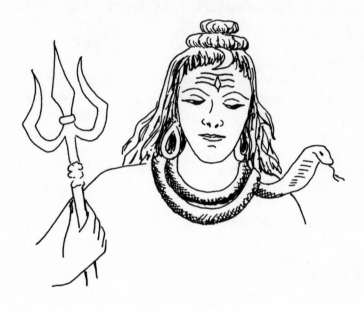

1. See page 14 for an illustration of the interplay of these aspects.

2. The yoga master B.K.S. Iyengar has developed this posture by separating it into several segments, with the emphasis on physical balance, a feeling of poise, quick movements such as jumping into the next phase, and correct focus.

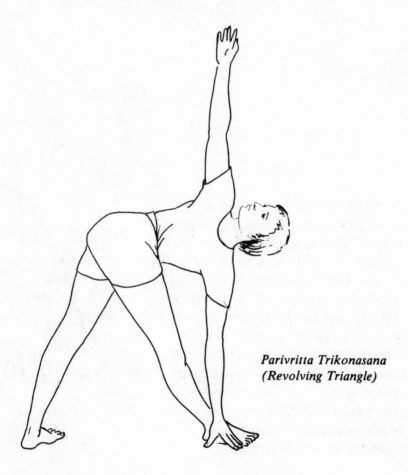

Parivritta Trikonasana
(Revolving Triangle)

Paschima means "the west." This pose stretches the western part of the body, which is the entire back from the head to the heels. From a sitting position with the legs extended straight out, the upper body stretches up from the pelvis, arms over the head. The upper body bends forward, the hands reaching toward the feet. Relaxing into the pose creates a sense of releasing into a place of surrender and humility.

paschimottanasana

SITTING FORWARD BEND

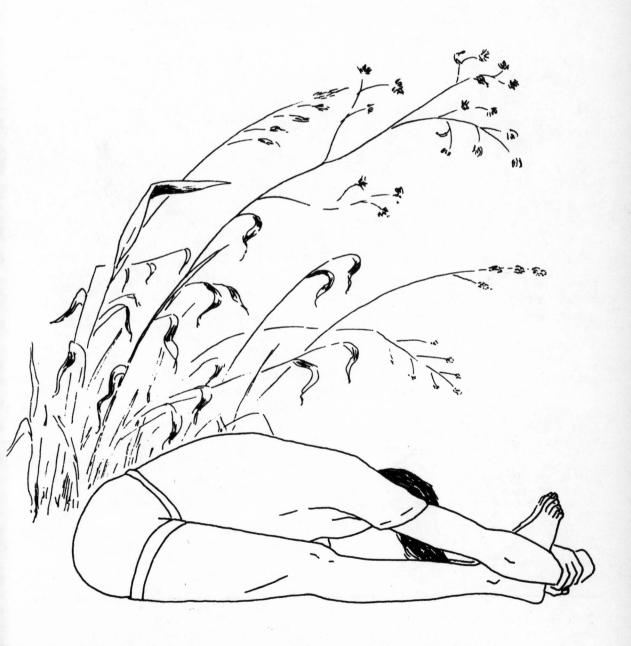

"Conscious effort on the back and visual effort in the front: brain and mind must function as one."

B.K.S. Iyengar

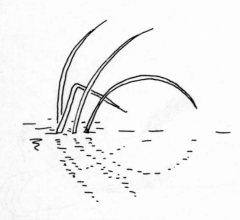

paschimottanasana

SITTING FORWARD BEND

W<small>HEN THE BODY</small> is bent forward from the hips, it is like folding it into halves, and sight is restricted. In Paschimottanasana it is as if there were a positive aspect in one's ability to execute the asana, and a negative aspect in one's limited vision. But these opposites are united at the hips, the point of bending.

Surrender is the important lesson that the asana teaches. There is a softening and an expansion from deep inside. Within the limited scope of movement in the body, this posture stretches muscles and ligaments; it stretches also the limitations in one's thinking, feeling, recognition, understanding. The surrender is particularly well expressed by the fact that one cannot see behind or above. In the acceptance of this situation lies humility. The hands, which are most expressive for a loving touch and secure holding, reach to grasp the feet, the foundation of being. In patience and surrender, then, we take the time to stretch and lengthen.

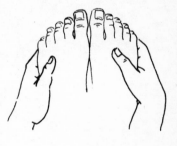

All asanas are intended to make the aspirant spine-conscious, and this one is no exception. Before one can fold with a straight spine, there is often a big hump, an obstacle that one has to get over in life. Only then is the surrender complete enough to make one receptive. Only then are the body, emotions, and mind strong enough to accept the insecurity of limited vision.

The Sanskrit word Paschimottanasana means "intense stretch to the west." In doing this posture the aspirant might think of the relevance of the west. What is the west? What does it mean in my life?

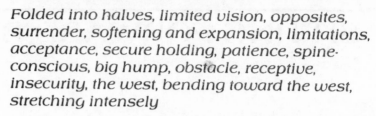

PASCHIMOTTANASANA:
Sitting Forward Bend Posture

Folded into halves, limited vision, opposites, surrender, softening and expansion, limitations, acceptance, secure holding, patience, spine-conscious, big hump, obstacle, receptive, insecurity, the west, bending toward the west, stretching intensely

To thrust forward to the ground brings awareness of the need to trust the innate divine nature. The intensity of the stretch and the recognition of limitations that must be overcome before it can be completed, instill humility again and again. At the center point where the bend begins, one becomes aware of the two halves of the body, the two halves of the mind. The opposites all through one's life and practice emerge with great clarity. It is in this clarity that insecurity vanishes. And, as one moves closer to perfection of the asana, one realizes—when standing up again—that turning back is impossible.

It is coming down to the ground, to the earth, that makes, not for the ending of life, but for a beginning. That deliberate action of surrender is the beginning of movement without and within, movement by which one advances on the Path. This asana is also one that is used for the practice of Brahmacharya.

PASCHIMOTTANASANA:
Sitting Forward Bend Posture

Thrust forward, the ground, trust, innate divine nature, intensity, humility, no turning back, center point, opposites, surrender, beginning of movement, positive and negative touch, separation, divided circle, answers within, inspiration, awe, wonder

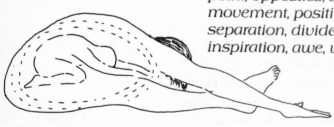

In Paschimottanasana, the upper body touches the lower, while the mind thinks in terms of higher and lower, peaceful and violent, positive and negative. Which is which? Can the separation of good and bad, like black and white, really be established? Can there really be a broken circuit of energy, or a divided circle? The answers—to be found within—will perhaps be an inspiration to bow down in awe and wonder at the Divine Wisdom that comes to the individual in so many ways.

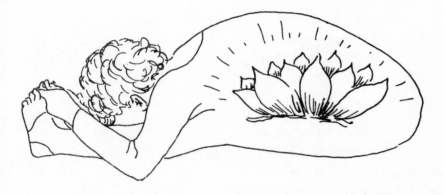

paschimottanasana   •*69*

SITTING FORWARD BEND

Ardha means "half." *Matsyendra* was a sage who spread the teachings of Yoga. In this pose, the right leg is on the floor and bent so that the foot is on the outside of the left buttock. The left leg is bent and upright with the foot on the outside of the right thigh. The body twists to the left with the right arm passed around the bent knee of the left leg, the hands clasped behind the back. The head turns to the left to look behind. The pose is repeated on the other side.

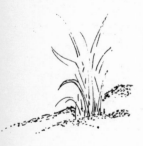
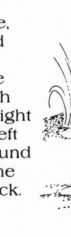
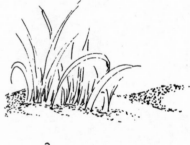

ardha matsyendrasana

SPINAL TWIST

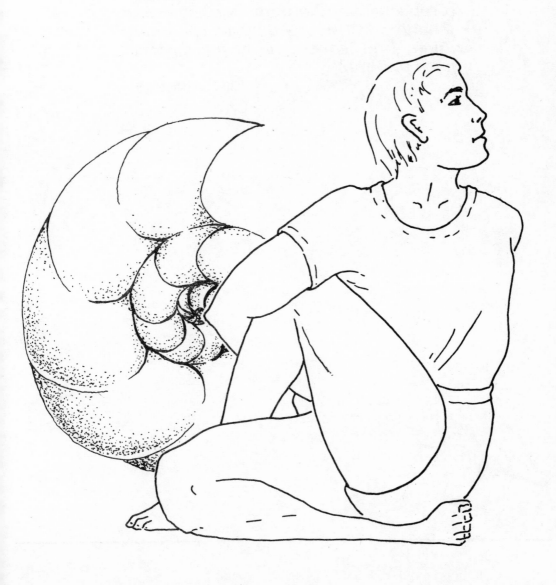

"The whole body, far from being ignored, is taken up in this spiritual alertness, till the whole man becomes pure flame. An alert, erect spine creates a spiritual intensity of concentration that burns out distracting thoughts and the brooding over past and future, and leaves one in the virginal fresh present."

B.K.S. Iyengar

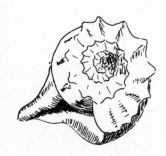

ardha matsyendrasana

SPINAL TWIST

IN ARDHA MATSYENDRASANA the body is twisted from a sitting position. The twisting of the spine touches on the basic foundation and functioning of the skeleton itself. A flexible mind and an inflexible spine can rarely be found together. If the body is tied in a knot, so are the mind and emotions. However, with sufficient depth of insight it can be recognized that what has been twisted can also be untwisted.

Concepts that are held rigidly will make the untwisting more difficult because of pride. Is it only the body that can twist in many different ways, or is this also the privilege of the mind? There is little that does not get twisted to some degree, however small—stories that we hear and retell, even the recording of dreams. Sometimes the mind is so flexible it can twist from "thine" to "mine" and "mine" to "thine."

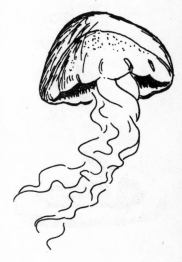

The twisting posture is a bit like a contorted spiral—a spiral being bent out of shape. Turning and twisting can come from the lower nature in oneself, from too many points of view that make one like a jellyfish, with no backbone. To untwist one's thinking so that things can be straight helps to unravel a variety of emotions that can twist one's true purpose.

To do this posture you must first come down from a standing position. You can think, How do I come down? What does it mean to sit on the ground? Am I "sitting on" a problem? Where did it begin? Can I go back to the basic event, before there was any bending and twisting? To unravel a problem you can go through each movement in the mind as you do in the asana.

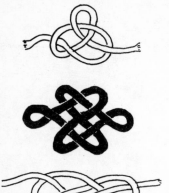

ARDHA MAṢYENDRASANA:
Spinal Twist Posture

Basic foundation, flexible, inflexible, tied in a knot,
mine and thine, contorted, bent out of shape,
turning and twisting, no backbone, twisted thinking,
points of view, sitting on a problem,
unravel a problem

Watching the body's ability to bend, and watching the untwisting of the bends, makes it easier to see the bending and twisting of the mind. You want the body to be flexible and supple; do you want your mind also to be flexible and supple? How flexible do you want to be? A person who is too flexible can be manipulated, almost invites manipulation; so one who is spineless must first firm up the spine, develop strength.

In doing the spinal twist you may find out that you do not listen, you do not see, you do not pay attention. Facts can be twisted for the sake of self-justification. A deliberately slow movement does not necessarily indicate that care has been taken, but rather it may be gaining time to twist the truth, to twist situations to get one's way, to be in control. And yet, at the same time, the twisting posture allows a different perspective. One's own personal development is a non-linear process. Who has not experienced in life the twist of events for the better?

The animal that can twist its body most easily is the snake, and its symbolism points to both wisdom and temptation. The twisting posture leads to introspection. But twisting can also be indicative of an indirect way of dealing with people—sometimes to escape criticism, sometimes just from habit.

Once the habit of twisting has been established, escaping from such mechanicalness will be rather difficult and take a lot of energy. But what a wonderful sense of freedom on getting out of the rut, on having loosened all this immobility—able once again to adapt!

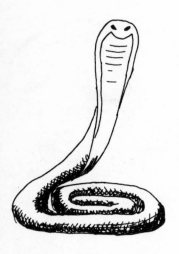

Pain or stiffness in the neck that was not discovered in any other asana is likely to appear here. Who gives me a pain in the neck? What gives me a stiff neck? What caused the shortening in the hamstrings and the hips? The tightness in these areas limits the body, but equally limits the mind. What immobilizes me, prevents me from adapting?

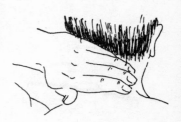

ARDHA MATSYENDRASANA:
Spinal Twist Posture

Manipulated, spineless, self-justification, twist the truth, be in control, different perspective, twist of events, indirect, escape criticism, habit, mechanicalness, freedom, stiff neck, pain in the neck, tightness, immobilized

Once the blocks that came about by twisting are removed, there is a change of perspective—seeing from a new angle. Looking back is no longer traumatic. To unwind and adjust not only affects the spine but also clears the vision. The twisting pose, stimulating introspection, should never be abandoned. It will be another step in ascending the mountain to freedom.

You may realize in your practice of this asana, that if you can twist so well for self-gratification—by twisting circumstances that surround you—you may also have twisted and veiled your true goal.

REFLECTIONS: Spinal Twist

The twist may be thought of as a spiral, the movement of which can go either upward or downward. The downward spiral will enmesh you in your lower nature, while the upward spiral will increase awareness and expand limitations.

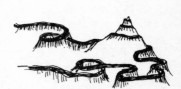

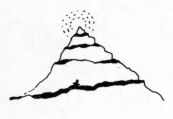

For the seeker who has an intense inner desire to pursue spiritual goals, the mind has to be bent and twisted in that direction. Social, cultural, and personal habits have to be bent to be overcome. Going into this posture is indicative of a decision to bend, and force a change in old ways of life to achieve the spiritual goal. These changes will manifest first in the personality and its various aspects. Sometimes the twisting or bending, as in a spiral, creates a tension that can be extremely useful. The release of stored energy is then available for a different use. Directing it into spiritual practices, such as Mantra, will allow the sincere aspirant to reach the goal.

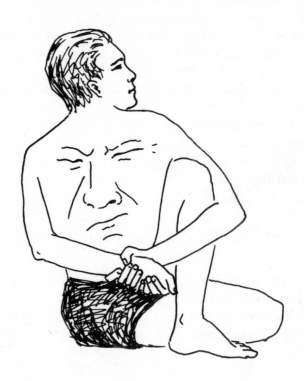

ardha matsyendrasana

TWIST

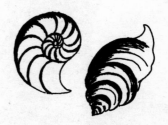

ardha matsyendrasana

TWIST

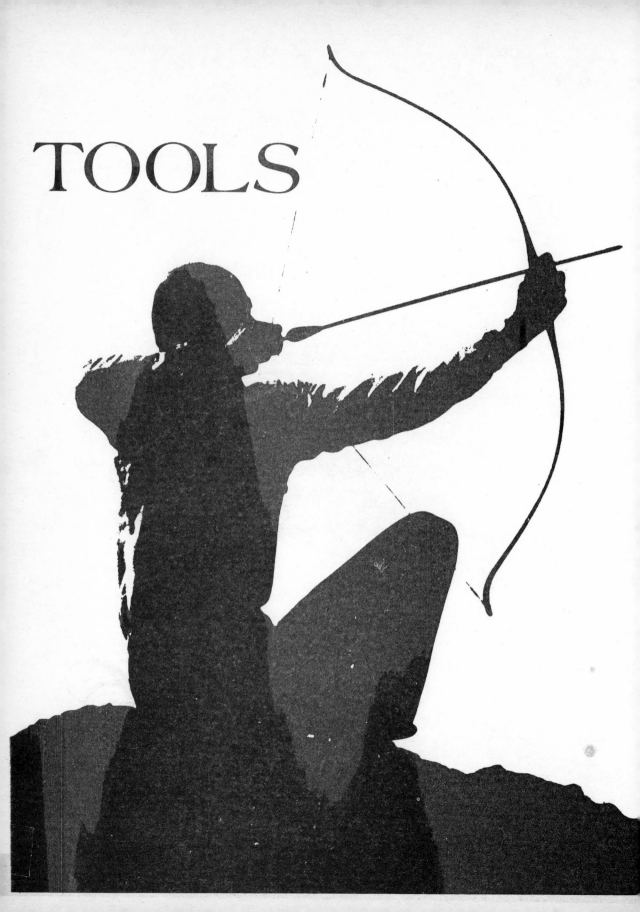

TOOLS

halasana

PLOUGH

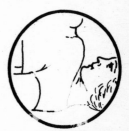

dhanurasana

BOW

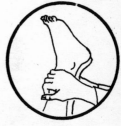

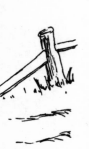

Hala means "plough." From a relaxed position lying down with the arms at the sides, the feet are brought over the head toward the ground. The arms and feet remain relaxed. The position suggests a plough.

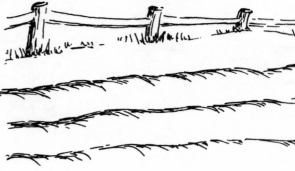

halasana
PLOUGH

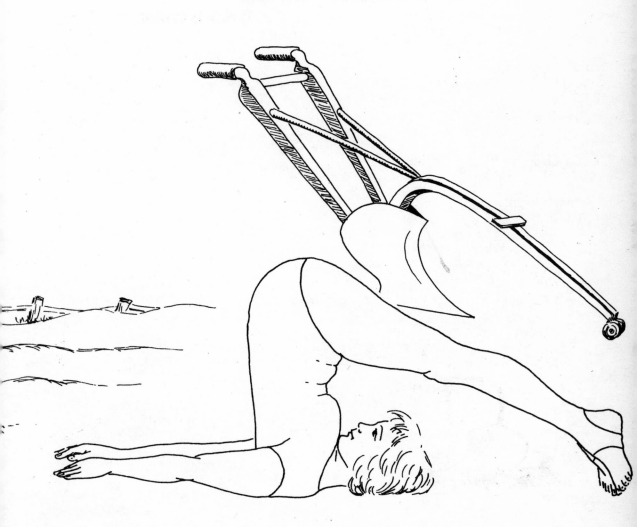

"You should be like a farmer: the day he sows, he is not happy thinking of the future harvest, he is happy to have planted well and to have sown well."

B.K.S. Iyengar

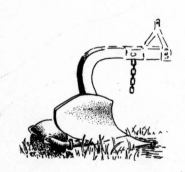

halasana

PLOUGH

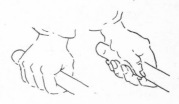

WHEN THE PLOUGH was made by hand it needed a strong grip, strong muscles, to break up the earth in preparation for fertilizing and seeding, to grow food for the nourishment of the people.

Bachofen, who wrote on the rights of mothers, has this to say about the plough: "The male ploughs open the womb of the earth and of the woman as well."[1] This compares the production of food with that of offspring, with the male ploughing open the womb of the female, breaking the hymen, to fertilize the womb in order to continue the species. [2]

To plough the earth, then, is to touch it with a rather violent touch,[3] breaking up the crust that may have formed for the protection of what is underneath. The harvesting of the fruits from the womb of the earth, and the birth of the baby from the womb of the mother, are also both violent acts.

Even surrender is not without a certain degree of violence because it often begins by sacrificing what is desired. The subduing of the self and of the self-will is always an act of violence. Friction between two opposites is the basis of life's continuum.

When you go into this posture think, What am I ploughing through in my life? What are the hard lumps I must break up? What do I want to plant in my ground? What do I really want to do? As I carry my legs back over my head, I feel constricted, yet secure. Is the security in my life constricting me?

HALASANA: Plough Posture

Strong grip, strong muscles, male ploughs the womb, seeding, violent, breaking up, protection, what is underneath? harvesting, fruits, child, birth, surrender, sacrifice, will, opposites

•83

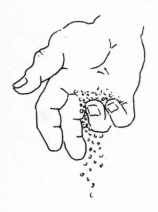

The *Bhagavad Gita* tells us that we should renounce the fruits of our labor, and dedicate them to the Divine. Perhaps the most difficult of these fruits to renounce are praise, recognition, fame, or wealth. We can also speak of ploughing the ground of life and making it fertile to receive the seeds of divine inspiration. The fruits of self-development that come from self-examination automatically become the fertilizer for further growth.

Even to sow the seeds of understanding, the ground of the mind must be ploughed. The weeds (concepts that have, like crab grass, grown deep) are hard to remove. The seeds of understanding can only grow in a fertile soil, one that is receptive, and in which the nourishment is of high quality. At the same time, discrimination is needed to distinguish good, healthy thoughts from the weeds of self-importance and fear— weeds that will crowd out the new growth. Discrimination can reveal what is truly inspiration, and what is still growing in the soil of self-will.

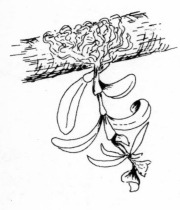

If we could plough our minds free of preconceived ideas, we would be free of convictions that served us well when we needed to survive in our world. Now that we have received the seed of divine inspiration, we may no longer want to cling with deep long roots to the earth. We may be ready to grow like an orchid, subsisting only on air and water, producing sufficient roots to cling to a surface like a tree, but not living off the tree—and producing delicate flowers of indescribable beauty. The flowers of inspiration also need space and freedom.

To plough the ground means holding the plough steady so the soil will turn over, making deep furrows, making deep cuts, and pulverizing the earth. As the earth has to be ploughed every year to keep it loose and aired, so the ground of the mind has to be ploughed over and over, to keep it open and receptive.

halasana

PLOUGH

The flowering process seems painful because obstacles must be removed from the mind. This is still within the control of the individual in spite of surrender to Teachings or Teacher. And like the earth whose furrow creates a separation, the practicing aspirant may often feel cut in the middle, separated into the physical and the spiritual selves. At such a moment, it is wise to consider that just as the earth is still whole beneath the furrow, so at a deeper level the two selves are still united.

In the process of watching one's own growth, as the spiritual plant unfolds, old desires may reappear, sometimes more powerfully than before. Since we do not want wild growth, we must harness—and direct toward the flower—the energy from emotions that are merely self-gratification in disguise.

The plough must always be kept in a perfect state of functioning; discrimination will become the share that must be kept sharp. Just as a farmer would not plough the land at night, so the aspirant must plough the mind and emotions in the light of cognizance and understanding. The work that has been done needs to be surveyed from time to time to assure oneself that it was done carefully. Too much moisture—too much emotion, too many tears—can make the ploughing difficult if not impossible.

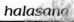

HALASANA: Plough Posture

Seeds, weeds, flowers, discrimination, deep furrows, deep cuts, open, receptive, orchid, preconceived ideas, convictions, between the physical and spiritual selves, look a little deeper, wild growth, harnessed

The aspirant will be constantly cultivating emotions, thinking, imagination, behavior toward others, as well as cultivating the body by doing the asanas. A careful attendance to dreams can be comforting as they will reveal what is still deep within the soil of the unconscious.

It is easy to become too optimistic after one's first attempt at ploughing. It is only repeated efforts that will turn up unseen hindrances. Emotions cannot be starved to death, but they can be channeled into a worship in which they find expression of a beneficial kind.

REFLECTIONS: Plough

In China, Egypt, and Peru the king blessed the work of the farmers and brought dignity to it by being the first one to touch the plough.[4] The ancients regarded agriculture as a religious art, and various gods and goddesses were invoked and worshipped to obtain a good harvest needed for the survival of the people. It is no surprise that the Buddha, coming from a small kingdom in northern India where agriculture prevailed and land and cattle represented wealth, used symbols and metaphors from nature to teach his disciples some important spiritual lessons. One day he took his disciples up to a hill, and pointing into the valley, said, "Look at the farmer, tilling first the good soil. Only when there is time and light left will he also take care of the second class field. He may not find time at all

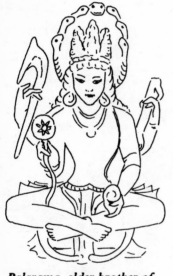

Balarama, elder brother of Krishna, holds the ploughshare.

for the third class of soil, or for anything thereafter." The same is true of aspirants; for the teacher to give time to the true seeker, who is represented as the good soil, makes sense.

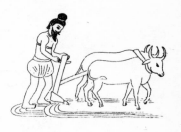

In another parable the Buddha said, "Faith is the seed; good works are the rain which makes it fruitful; wisdom and meekness are the parts of the plough." He also said, "The mind is the reins and diligence is the patient ox [cow]."[5] There is a similarity between the Buddha's parable and the pre-Christian Yoke of Wisdom: "Put your neck under the yoke and let your soul receive instruction: she is hard at hand to find. . . . Work your work betimes and in his time he will give you your reward."[6]

In the East there are many delightful stories that help the spiritual seeker to remember the duties as well as the taboos.[7] The field is the Dharma; the weeds are the clinging worldly existence; the plough is the way to wisdom, to sowing and reaping imperishable fruits.[8] If purity could be a seed one could sow, and if all efforts and attentions could be directed toward the work that is performed, then the harvest, accordingly, would be just one step from Nirvana. The old has to be destroyed before the new can come. The old ego, all the old personality aspects that clamor for attention, creating obstacles, has to be destroyed to make room for the new growth. The hard crust of greed, revenge, mercilessness, deafness, has to be broken up so that the seeds of understanding and compassion can be sown; and so that the fruit of the true Self, a heart full of love and devotion, a mind receptive to Divine Wisdom, can be enjoyed.

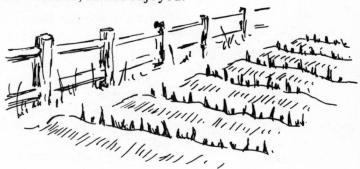

halasana

PLOUGH

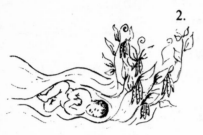

1. Bachofen, *Myth, Religion & Mother Right*, 191-192.

2. "The concept of the earth as both bearing and nourishing mother has been extremely prominent in the mythologies both of hunting societies and of planters. . . . According to the planters, it is in the mother's body that the grain is sown; the plowing of the earth is a begetting and the growth of the grain a birth." Campbell, *The Masks of God: Primitive Mythology*, 66.

   In some cultures women were involved symbolically in the act of ploughing. "Women are sometimes supposed to be able to make rain by ploughing, or pretending to plough. Thus the Pshaws and Chewsurs of the Caucasus have a ceremony called 'ploughing the rain,' which they observe in time of drought. Girls yoke themselves to a plough and drag it into a river, wading in the water up to their girdles." Similar traditions were found in Armenia, Transylvania, the Caucasian province of Georgia, and parts of India. Fraser, *The Golden Bough*, 92-93.

3. "Ploughing signifies the breaking of the original prima materia into the multiplicity of creation; the opening of the earth to the influence of heaven; man's mastery over the earth; fertility. The plough is phallic and the ploughshare impregnates the earth; the furrow is feminine. In North American Indian and other nomadic traditions ploughing is evil and a violation of the body of the Mother Earth." Cooper, *Illustrated Encyclopaedia of Traditional Symbols*, 133.

4. In China, "grain culture is of such importance in the national life that the Emperor used to set the example to the people every spring by means of a ceremonial ploughing of a sacred field with a highly ornamental plough kept for the purpose." Williams, *Outlines of Chinese Symbolism*, 1.

5. Bayley, *Lost Language of Symbolism*, part 2, 258.

6. Ibid., 256.

7. The plough is also seen in legends of the East as a tool for revealing hidden treasures. A story in the *Ramayana* illustrates this. Janaka, a king dedicated to the principles and practices of Karma Yoga, uncovered a beautiful baby girl as he was ploughing the earth in the sacrifical ground. He adopted the baby and named her Sita. She later became the wife of Rama.

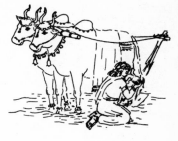

8. The plough as a way to wisdom is illustrated in the life of Milarepa, a Tibetan yogi who achieved Self-realization in one lifetime by disciplining his mind through hard work, perseverance, and rigorous spiritual practice. His Guru spoke of his potential: "Thy drinking up of all the *chhang* which I there gave thee, and thy ploughing up the field entirely, predicted that thou wouldst be a worthy *shishya* who would imbibe the whole of the Spiritual Truths which I had to impart to thee." Evans-Wentz, *Tibet's Great Yogi Milarepa,* 133.

When Milarepa was very discouraged about his lack of progress he had the following dream: "I was engaged in ploughing a very stiff and hardened plot of land, which defied all mine efforts; and despairing of being able to plough it, was thinking of giving up the task. Thereupon, my beloved Guru Marpa appeared in the heavens and exhorted me, saying 'Son, put forth thine energy and persevere in the ploughing; thou are sure to succeed, despite the hardness of the soil.' Then Marpa himself guided the team; the soil was ploughed quite easily; and the field produced a rich harvest." Ibid., 188.

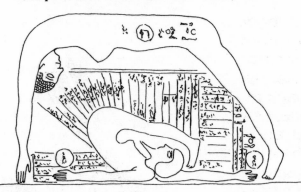

The Egyptian sky goddess, Nut, bends over the figure of Geb, the Earth, who seems to perform the plough posture as he revolves upon himself.

halasana

PLOUGH

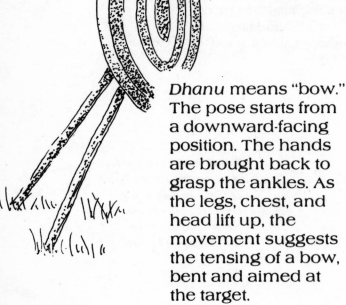

Dhanu means "bow." The pose starts from a downward-facing position. The hands are brought back to grasp the ankles. As the legs, chest, and head lift up, the movement suggests the tensing of a bow, bent and aimed at the target.

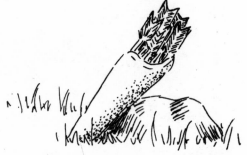

dhanurasana
BOW

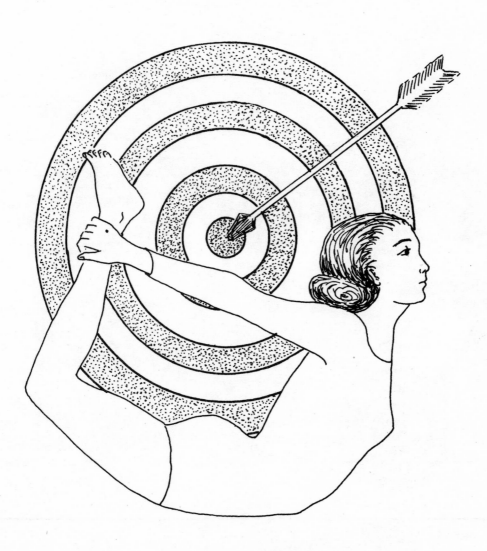

"Singularity of purpose should be your aim."

B.K.S. Iyengar

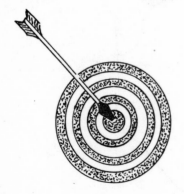

dhanurasana

BOW

In Japan, ARCHERY is treated with such reverence that it is almost a religion. D. T. Suzuki, in the introduction to Eugen Herrigel's *Zen and the Art of Archery,* says that the practice of archery is meant to train the mind.[1] The hitter and the hit become one reality, no longer opposing objects. Students receive careful training and preparation and it is, therefore, used as a means toward a spiritual goal. In the art of archery, as in Zen, great emphasis is put on breathing. Tension and holding the breath, releasing and exhaling, are finely attuned. The idea that one has to be the doer at all costs because nothing would happen otherwise, is an obstacle to be overcome in archery as in all of life.

The bow has many uses besides sending the arrow to its target. The bow of a saw is under similar stress when at work. But the delicacy of the bow of the violin, and its peculiar use, shows the great complexity and enormous variety of human functions.

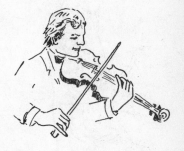

It takes great effort to assess the many targets that are available, the variety of tensions that have to be imposed on the bow, and the different aims for the arrow. The purpose of the arrow is to fly straight and true to the target.[2] The purpose of the bow also needs clear definition. One is useless without the other. And what is the target? Is there a target, a larger one, in the distance, with many intermediate ones along the way? Is the main target well-defined, clear? What is represented by the concentric circles of a target? Considerations such as these indicate the sensitivity and strength needed in the handling and the tensing of the bow. Those who have achieved mastery of these two—strength and sensitivity—have also achieved swiftness.

DHANURASANA: Bow Posture

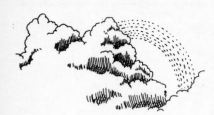

Practice, careful training, spiritual goal, breathing, holding, releasing, fine tuning, the doer, stress, delicacy, complexity, many targets, variety of tensions, different aims, sensitivity, strength, swiftness; feeling stretched, pressure on my solar plexus, don't feel very well-tuned, what am I aiming for?

The bow that is most admired and gazed upon with wonder is the rainbow, best known for its mention in the Bible. We are told in Genesis, "And God said, I do set my bow in the cloud, and it shall be for a token of a covenant between me and the earth. And it shall come to pass, when I bring a cloud over the earth, that the bow shall be seen in the cloud."[3] This promise, although perhaps dimly remembered, may underlie the feeling of hope and optimism that seeing a rainbow usually evokes. Even in Islam, where little symbolism is used, the power of God and his connection with human life is represented by the bow: "The grip of the bow in the middle, uniting both parts, is the union of Allah with Mohammed."[4]

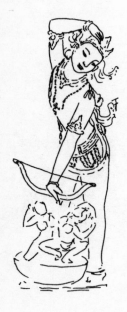

The bow and arrow were originally instruments for warfare. But in East Indian philosophy the warfare of Kama, the god of love, is of a different kind. He wants to shoot the heart and imbue love in that target, so the continuation of life may be secured. He carries a very special bow that has flowers and colorful ribbons attached; and yet the bow is the god himself. The five arrows of Kama, "whose arrows are flowers,"[5] are also connected with the noose and the hook in rituals for producing love and surrender. Kama has a miniaturized Western counterpart in Cupid.

The heart as the target suggests that there can be sweetness in pain. The function of Kama is to ensure the continuation of life. One who does not wish to be on the receiving end of Kama's arrows may have to break the bow, symbolizing the point of departure from attachment, sensuality, and desire. In an Indian legend Lord Krishna broke the bow, which is described as being of the size of a rainbow and equally colorful. It broke the moment Lord Krishna tried to string it. And the sound of the break thundered throughout the heavens.[6]

The archer can be seen as an active intelligence, drawing on divine inspiration as well as on his own physical strength and skill. Rama-chandra,[7] one of the popular Hindu gods, is shown with the bow in his left hand. These ancient symbols can be an inspiration for the aspirant to delve deeper into the meaning of Dhanurasana.

To meet all the conditions of this asana demands flexibility, a limber spine. But flexibility has to be balanced with strength. The tension and relaxation that are necessary produce an interplay of forces, and cannot be separated from each other. If bending forward as in Paschimottanasana has to be counterbalanced with bending backward as in Dhanurasana, we are reminded that one has both within oneself—the flexibility and relaxation (humility and surrender) of the forward bend and the strength and tension of the back bend. How far should one bend? When is enough truly enough?

DHANURASANA: Bow Posture

Rainbow, covenant, promise, warfare, Cupid, love, attachment, sensuality, desire, breaking the bow, active intelligence, flexibility, limber spine, strength, tension, relaxation, bending backward, counterbalance

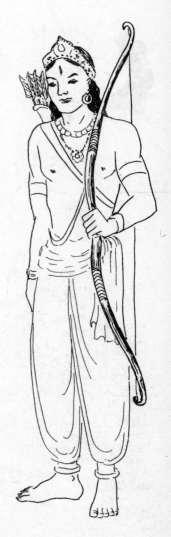

Sometimes we feel that destiny, or the Divine, tenses our bow to the breaking point, and we may desperately pray for release without realizing that our limitations are self-inflicted. Letting go of the judgment about ourselves is very difficult. Yet, at the same time, for the sake of acceptance from others, we will bend over backward, although not without grudging having to do so. However, bending over backward for the sake of reconciliation, for peace and harmony, may sometimes be the right thing to do.

The bow posture is like a bowl into which can be put much goodness that is nourishing on many levels. It is like the first half of the circle of perfection that will be completed in time. It is accepting the opposite position—bringing together the head and feet in the reverse manner—so that the exposed throat, the seat of self-will, becomes very vulnerable. Symbolically, the bow is masculine and feminine at the same time, unifying the opposites of strength and flexibility, tension and surrender.

REFLECTIONS: Bow

In a Chinese story, Yi,[8] the Excellent Archer who shot down nine suns, could do so because he had a magic bow. It seems that the bow and the arrow are inseparable, and that the clarity attained by the proper discrimination, decision, and pursuit of a spiritual goal, will lead to an almost magical power.

In Hinduism, the mystic syllable OM is the bow, the arrow is the mind, and the Higher Self (Brahma) is the mark. Unwavering concentration is the action. Penetration of the target by the arrow is the achievement.[9] The recognition of what needs to be done to achieve this experience is overwhelming, and this is expressed by Arjuna in the First Discourse of the *Bhagavad Gita* when he says:

28. Seeing these, my kinsmen, O Krishna, arrayed,
    eager to fight,
29. My limbs fail and my mouth is parched, my body
    quivers and my hair stands on end,
30. The (bow) Gandiva slips from my hand, and also
    my skin burns all over; I am unable even to
    stand, and my mind is reeling, as it were.[10]

As Arjuna later understands, his friends and relatives are his own personality aspects that have to be killed before he can progress spiritually. And attachment, which is often mistaken for love, must also be overcome in order to achieve the needed concentration.

Lord Indra's elusive bow is referred to in the Mantra for the Manipura Chakra, dealing with the sense of sight and the emotions. The following commentary is given in *Kundalini: Yoga for the West:*

> The rainbow has no substance, it is intangible and
>   cannot be grasped.
> The rainbow is an optical illusion which becomes
>   perceptible to the sense of sight under certain
>   conditions.
> Sometimes the mind builds a rainbow to another
>   dimension.
> Sometimes flashes of lightning (insights) glitter with
>   jewels of intuition.
> Who can gaze at the sun when it is at the zenith?
> The light, too great, too blinding, will scorch the mind.
> The dark cloud offers much-needed rest, time to gather
>   new strength.[11]

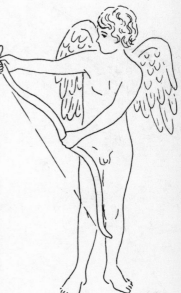

How much more inspiring is the thought of Indra's bow than the playfulness of Kama trying, like Cupid, to shoot his arrows at the heart! It is Kama, the god of love, who tries to detract human beings from the deeper love for the Divine, ensnaring them in attachments—attachments that always have their price, ending at some point in pain.

As Kahlil Gibran says in *The Prophet,* "Your children are not your children. They are the sons and daughters of Life's longing for itself. . . . You are the bows from which your children as living arrows are sent forth. . . . Let your bending in the archer's hand be for gladness; for even as He loves the arrow that flies, so He loves also the bow that is stable." [12]

This is the kind of love that the Venerable Nagasena speaks about when he tells King Milinda that the aspirant, in order to be in accord with other aspirants, needs to learn to bend like "a well-made and balanced bow [which] bends equally from end to end and does not resist stiffly like a post."[13]

dhanurasana

BOW

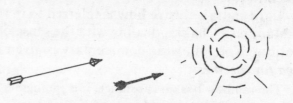

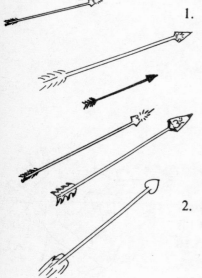

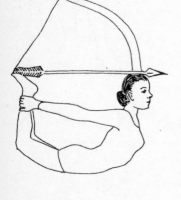

1. Herrigel, *Zen in the Art of Archery,* vi. Herrigel writes that the "aim consists in hitting a spiritual goal, so that fundamentally the marksman aims at himself and may even succeed in hitting himself. . . . Archery is still a matter of life and death to the extent that it is a contest of the archer with himself. In this contest . . . is revealed the secret essence of this art. . . . The more obstinately you try to learn how to shoot the arrow for the sake of hitting the goal, the less you will succeed in the one and the further the other will recede. What stands in your way is that you have a much too willful will. You think that what you do not do yourself does not happen." Ibid., 4, 5, 34.

2. "The flight of our spiritual arrow is a flight and an emergence from a total darkness underground and the chiaroscuro of space under the Sun into realms of spiritual Light where no Sun shines, nor Moon, but only the Light of the Spirit, which is Its own illumination." *Coomaraswamy. I: Selected Papers,* 447.

3. *The Holy Bible,* Genesis 9:13-14. This bow represents the higher mind and is a link between God and man.

4. Cooper, *Illustrated Encyclopaedia of Traditional Symbols,* 24.

5. Zimmer, *Philosophies of India,* 140.

6. The reader who is interested in the many facets of Lord Krishna should consult the Bibliography for sources of Hindu mythology.

7. Rama is known as the destroyer of the wicked.

8. *Larousse,* 278. For other stories involving the bow, see Tawney, *Ocean of Story,* vol. 4, and the *Mahabharata.* Of particular interest in the *Mahabharata* is a story illustrating the importance of conquering the mind rather than external enemies. A

royal sage named Alarka, "having with his bow conquered this world as far as the ocean, having peformed very difficult deeds, turned his mind to subtle [subjects]. Alarka said: 'my mind is become too strong; that conquest is constant in which the mind is conquered. Though surrounded by enemies, I shall direct my arrows elsewhere. . . . I will cast very sharp-edged arrows at the mind.'" "The Anugita," 296.

9. *Mundaka Upanishad,* 2.2:4.

In the Buddhist tradition the bow represents willpower. "The bow is the mind which dispatches the arrows of the 5 senses." Cooper, *Illustrated Encyclopaedia of Traditional Symbols,* 24.

10. *Bhagavad Gita,* 1:28-30.

In certain religious ceremonies the bow symbolizes the killer of enemies. *Satapatha Brahmana,* part III:5, 3.

Another Hindu myth which tells of the strength needed to bend a special bow in order to win a divine treasure is the story of how Rama won Sita in marriage. See Coomaraswamy, *Myths of the Hindus and Buddhists,* 28.

11. Sivananda Radha, *Kundalini: Yoga for the West,* 308.

12. Gibran, *The Prophet,* 17-18.

13. *The Questions of King Milinda,* VII, I, 18.

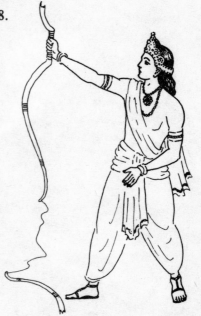

King Janaka decreed that no one would win his daughter Sita in marriage who could not handle a special bow that was so heavy it took 500 men to move it. Rama picked up the bow with ease and as he strung it, it broke, cracking like thunder.

dhanurasana

BOW

PLANTS

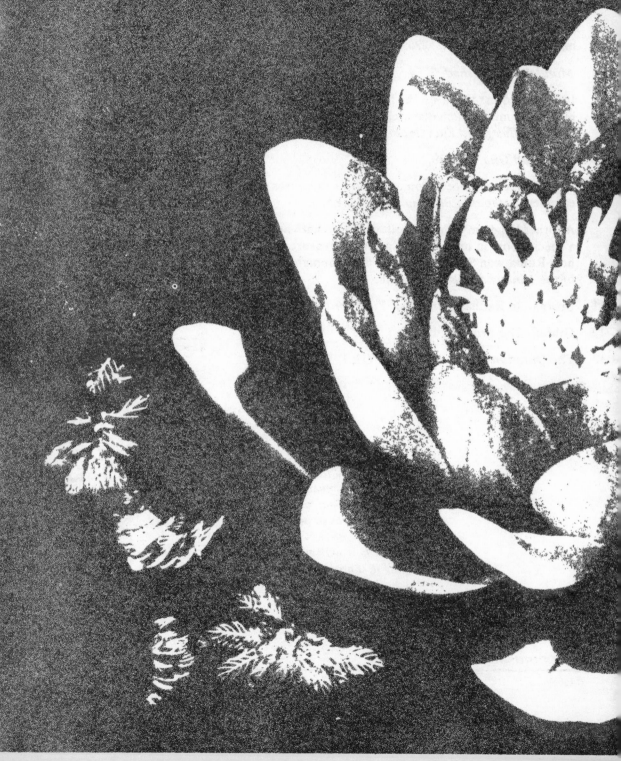

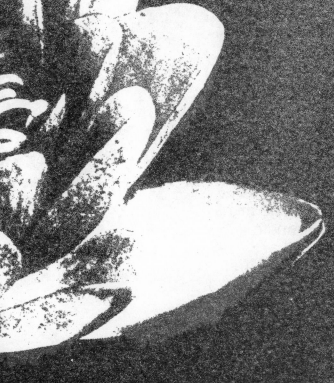

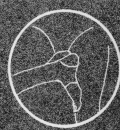
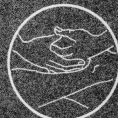

vrikshasana
TREE

padmasana
LOTUS

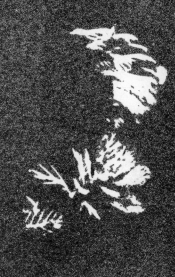

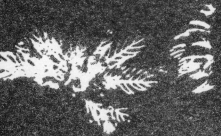

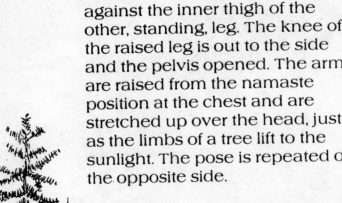

Vriksha means "tree." In this posture, a steady, rooted stance is created by bringing one foot against the inner thigh of the other, standing, leg. The knee of the raised leg is out to the side and the pelvis opened. The arms are raised from the namaste position at the chest and are stretched up over the head, just as the limbs of a tree lift to the sunlight. The pose is repeated on the opposite side.

vrikshasana

TREE

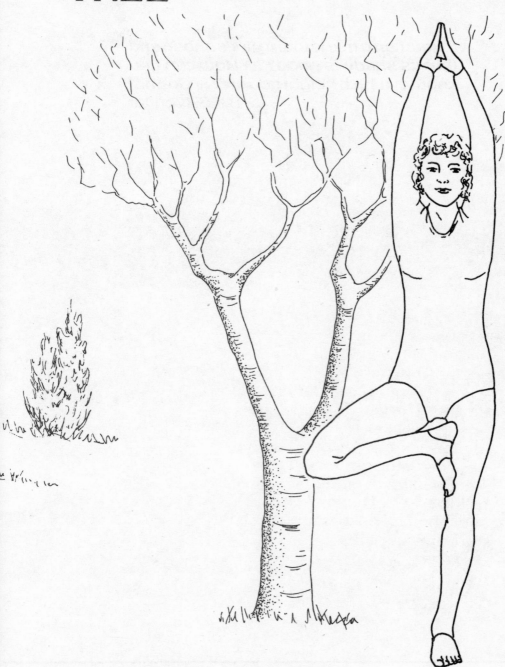

"How can a tree know it gives shade and that its shade is good? . . . How can you know at which height you are? . . . Go on."

B.K.S. Iyengar

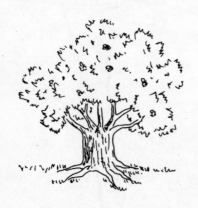

vrikshasana

TREE

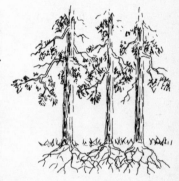

IF WE LOOK AT A TREE, the two things we see first are the large trunk and the crown. What comes to mind?—the alignment, the uprightness, the strength. The trees of the forest have always been able to hold themselves up without the support of fences or posts. There is a balance between the spread of the branches of the crown, and the root system which expands in width and in depth, reaching to assimilate nutrients. To think of this evokes a feeling of mystery. How does the water rise upward from the roots to nourish the branches in their very tops?

As you do this posture, questions such as these might arise in your mind: Where have my roots spread? Where do they get their nourishment? Which are mine and which belong to someone else? What competes with my roots for nourishment?

The importance of the tree to mankind since the beginning of time, physically and spiritually, is shown in legends of ancient civilizations. The myths surrounding the tree indicate that as far back as the old Sumerians, people were seeking to discover the secrets of life, of a greater power beyond their ordinary sense perceptions. In one of their myths, the Sumerians speak of a tree as being a temple, a bond between heaven and earth.[1] The ancient Chinese believed that the souls of the gods reside in trees; thus trees were sacred for them also.

The great Egyptian god Ra appeared in the morning between two sycamore trees of beautiful turquoise color. The sycamores were sacred because it was believed that some deities such as the goddesses Nut and Hathor—beings who were no longer in heaven but who were not touching the ground—lived in the tree tops. They were the bridge between the upper and lower worlds.

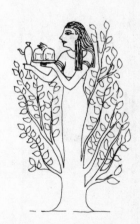

The sky goddess, Nut

The aspirant stands in just such a relationship, symbolized by this posture.[2] Recognition of the powerful symbol the tree

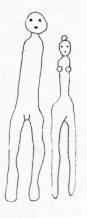

has been for cultures the world over helps one to rise above self-importance and achieve a different perspective on life.[3]

In *Myths of Creation,* Phillip Freund has tried to find an explanation for the strenuous search of human beings to understand these mysteries of life. He tells us that the Yana Indians in California created their tribe by whispering secret words over sticks which were made to stand up, and which then became men and women. In Scandinavia, the origin of human life is told in stories of the Edda. In this myth, two trees were found and carved into a man and a woman, who were then given spirit and life and declared to be the parents of mankind.[4] Often in myths, figures carved from wood are brought to life by the rhythm and sounds of a drum.[5]

In some cultures, woman was formed from the branches of the tree; and sometimes the gods, incapable of dealing with loneliness, formed a wife out of a tree. It is interesting to see how great is the sadness of even the male god when he realizes he is alone.

The oak has probably the greatest significance in the myths of the West as it represents the main residence of the supreme god. No sacred rites were performed by the Gauls without oak leaves, and Socrates is supposed to have sworn by the oak as a sacred oracle tree.[6] The oak was also a place of security, and Homer reports that rulers made agreements there that would influence the destiny of their people.

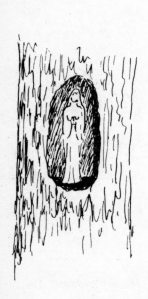

When Christianity expanded into the corners of Europe, statues of the Virgin were nestled into hollows in oak trees. In this way, the old and the new were combined. The new cannot take place without the old; one always builds on what is already there. In spite of the forward movement of Christianity, the influence of those early days remained. Knights made their pacts under an oak tree, letting blood from their veins spill into a vessel where it would mix, and then dedicating it to the oak tree. Here, letting blood is symbolic of letting go of accusations and criticism, and surrendering to the oak tree, a symbol of masculine strength. Surrender and masculine strength need to be united to attain power beyond the usual human experience.

The rich symbolism of the myths connected with the tree can enhance the understanding of oneself and one's place in the world, bridging the realms above and below. As you stand in this posture, personalize this mythology by thinking of the meaning of words such as the ones in the following list.

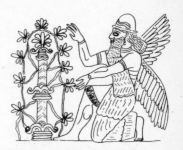

Assyrian deity with sacred tree
(900 BC)

VRIKSHASANA: Tree Posture

Alignment, uprightness, without support, balance, root system, secrets of life, greater power, temple, heaven and earth, sacred rites, letting blood, letting go—of accusations, criticism; surrendering, masculine strength, nourishment

Trees, like people, have their destiny, and much of the survival of the tree depends on the sturdiness of the trunk and the branches, sturdiness that must be balanced with flexibility. The oak tree breaks in a storm, while the willow swings back from the force of the wind. Am I unyielding like the oak, or can I bend with the forces of destiny?

Bark covers the trunk like a garment, protecting it from the weather, splitting from the winds and temperature changes. As the tree grows it puts on layer after layer, only to split over and over again. What is the rough garment that covers me? What conditions does it protect me from?

The circumference of the tree indicates the space that the roots take up: as above, so below. A cross-section of one of the mighty redwood trees or a ponderosa pine will reveal the story of its life, like a daily diary. It tells of normal growth, of times of drought, and of neighboring trees that competed with it for nourishment. It gives the scientist much information of the past; daily reflection jotted down in a diary can give me much information about my past, my interactions with others, my growth—normal or stunted.

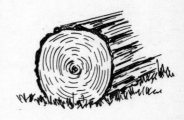

The cyclical nature of the tree in its growth through the various seasons is like the seasons of human life and its process of growth. There is competition among trees as there is among people; destiny places stones, rocks, and gravel in the soil of

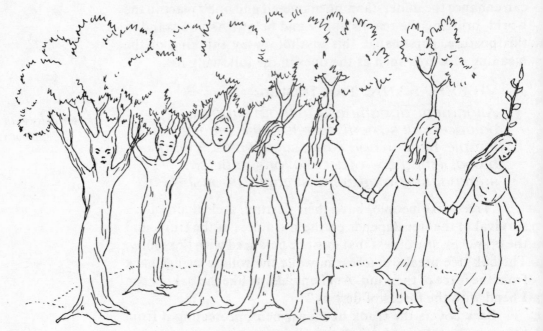

Tree women progressively detaching themselves from the vegetable kingdom

both trees and humans. With trees, the competition is in the struggle for survival. But in many people it has gone beyond survival to greed, greed that bears the signs of the decay of health and growth. When the leaves cover the ground in their enchanting colors, from a subtle yellow to a deep red, they are already dead. There is beauty in death, in the promise of new life to follow. But in human life, the dead leaves resemble personality aspects from the very subtle to the gross and flashy. When greed has bred on "success," then the personality aspects, like the leaves, though brilliant in color, show that growth has stopped and the process of decay has begun. Dried up tree tops tell that the fate of the tree has been sealed, that its destiny of death will soon arrive.

In some cultures, if fruit trees do not bear fruit, the farmer will take an ax and threaten them by cutting off unproductive branches. Perhaps the pruning of fruit trees in our culture is another way of doing the same thing. The result is usually increased yield. The aspirant must also prune branches that are not productive, and cut away side growth.

Trees are sometimes cut down just for firewood, to serve the comfort of human beings. Others are turned into furniture, and although people admire the wonderful lines and grain, there is no concern about the tree from which the wood came. Some trees are cut into boards to build houses and shelters, and the wood absorbs the vibrations of the humans who live in them. Emotions may range from sorrow to violent anger. Some trees have wood that inspires the carver to produce pieces of art; the wood then has to bear prickings, chippings, and poundings. What are we sacrificing that is worth preserving in ourselves, for the sake of comfort and worldly success?

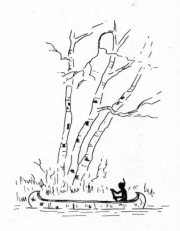

The tree has to surrender to the raindrops that fall on it, and its bare branches carry inches of cold and icy snow. Wherever the tree is, it must share. When it is large enough the birds build their nests in it with firm attachment. Likewise, the aspirant must cling to the Divine with firm attachment. Trees carry the weight of many creatures: animals like the bear or tiger, as well as the snake, the worm, or the little bug. I must carry my past, my mistakes, my forgetfulness, my habits of criticism, pride, and resentment.

The tree is in constant interaction with the earth from which it draws nutrients, and it is in interaction with the air that flows in powerful or gentle currents from the north to the south or from the west to the east. In the currents of human destiny each individual must hold his or her ground, being well-rooted, not in earth but in heaven, finding the balance in the relationship between reason and intuition.

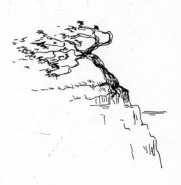

VRIKSHASANA: Tree Posture

Destiny, sturdiness, flexibility, oak and willow, protective bark, seasons of human life, competition, struggle for survival, greed, beauty in death, promise of new life, success, decay, personality aspects, pruning, comfort, sacrificing, share, firm attachment, carry: my past, mistakes, resentment; interaction, rooted in heaven, reason, intuition

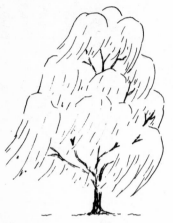

All those interacting influences demand both surrender and constant adjustment. The oak must be strong, yet not too inflexible; the willow must be flexible, yet not allow itself to be beaten to the ground by all the whims of destiny. The tree has no choices; but the aspirant, in facing the many currents of destiny, has the power of choice and the ability to discriminate.

REFLECTIONS: Tree

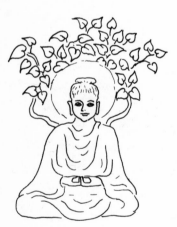

Joseph Campbell, in his *Primitive Mythology,* speaks of the great Cosmic Tree.[7] At its root is a guardian serpent and on its top branches sits an eagle. There is a distinct difference between the tree in the Garden of Eden, giving to human beings the knowledge of good and evil, and this Eastern Tree of Creation, which is a tree of the world, nourishing all mankind.

Prince Gautama found Liberation while meditating under the Bodhi tree, the tree of enlightenment, the tree of wisdom.[8] This world-tree is also described in the *Bhagavad Gita,* XV:1-2:

1. They (the wise) speak of the indestructible peepul tree having its root above and branches below, whose leaves are the metres or hymns: he who knows it is a knower of the Vedas.

2. Below and above spread its branches, nourished by the Gunas; sense-objects are its buds; and below, in the world of men, stretch forth the roots, originating action.

The Tree of Life occurs often in Zoroastrian theology, and the *Kabbalah* also speaks of a sacred tree that embodies many secrets, ancient mystical traditions. Some Muslims claim that Paradise has many trees with many leaves, and that the name of a human being, when it is born, is written on each leaf. The tree, then, is like the book of life. I have known families who would plant a tree every time a child was born, or others who would plant a tree in memory of a member of the family who died.

A fascinating Egyptian painting of the thirteenth century B.C. showed the mother goddess distributing food and drink from the branches of the Tree of Life.[9] In fact, she is part of this tree. The twice-seven branches of an East Indian tree, fashioned from bronze in a delicate manner, emerge from a central axis which is the seat of the lotus-sun, source of all life. The tree of divine life spreads throughout the universe and gives shelter to all sorts of creatures on its branches and under its leaves. Its divine message can only be perceived by intuition.

Nordic life was united by the great ash, Esche, also called Igdrasio. "The way it [the tree] is connected with all parts of the universe, all aspects of life, make it one of the most original creations of Nordic mythology."[10] Because of its deep roots it was symbolic of bridging the underworld and the realms of humanity, and also sometimes the realms of heroes and gods. Three of its mighty roots are of particular importance: there is one that grows deep to the fountain (water table), nourishing all beings; another is the texture that is woven from the threads of life and nature; and wisdom claims the third root. But snakes and deer are permitted to feed on the roots, bark, and leaves of the great ash, because the deer is symbolic of spiritual experiences and the snake of wisdom. On the top of this

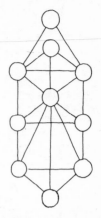

The Kabbalistic tree

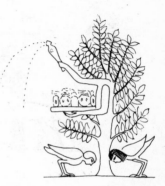

Egyptian mother goddess

vrikshasana

TREE

gigantic tree the eagle is joined by a cock and a hawk to keep
watch and to warn the gods should enemies approach.

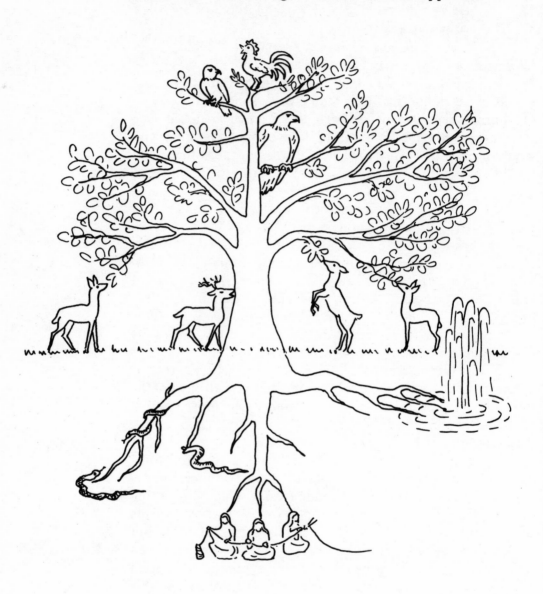

vrikshasana

TREE

In Scandinavia a story survives that tells about the destruction of the world; it was only due to the survival of a few humans that the future of mankind was secured. They were hidden in the trunk of Yggdrasill, the world-tree, which was immune to fire, flame, and darkness. These human beings could live on the morning dew until the earth was resurrected by Balder, the god of light. "For the new world, unlike the old, was not under threat of catastrophe.... 'The black dragon has fled far away and the shining serpent has left the depths of the pit.'" [11]

The shining serpent symbolizes the gift of prophecy that is received when one grows into the Light, defeating the black dragon of egoism. Survival is, then, overcoming the adversities one experiences in life.

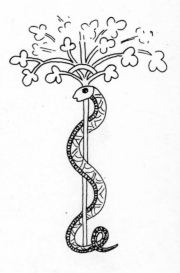

Many trees have leaves and bark that have healing and medicinal properties. Trees also symbolize other kinds of healing; to bring a branch of the olive tree means peace. [12] And, of course, there is the wooden cross on which Jesus was nailed. [13] But the palm tree is also connected with him, and means victory over death. In the symbolism of the Christmas tree, greenness stands for life and its sacredness, and the ever-presence of the Life Force or God. The lights on the tree are symbolic for the Light in us that needs to be renewed by the oil of aspiration. Evergreen trees are a reassurance that wisdom is ever ready, ever alive, and thereby available to those who have the inclination to apply it. [14]

A tree can only grow strong and healthy in an environment that suits its needs. But the tree cannot pull up its roots. It had no choice where the seed fell from which it grew. Aspirants may have to pull up all roots to find an environment that will support proper development; they may even have to create their own "heaven." The aspirant has no choice but to struggle for survival, health, strength, and harmony. Everything hinges on the Tree of Knowledge.

The sage Nagasena, when answering King Milinda's questions, said: The first quality of the tree that an aspirant should have is to bear the flowers of emancipation and the fruits of Samanaship,[15] as the tree bears fruits and flowers. The second is, as a tree casts its shadow over the men who come to it, and stay beneath it, just so should the aspirant receive with kindness, both as regards their bodily wants and their religious necessities, those that wait upon him, and remain near him. The third is, as the tree makes no distinction in the shadow it affords, so the aspirant should make no distinction, treating all with kindness.[16]

Trees of a similar kind are found in clusters. They stand together. Spiritual people are wise to stand together—communicating, chanting, meditating under a tree.

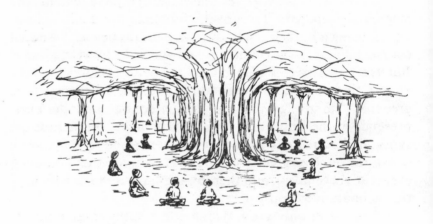

Banyen tree

1. The original symbolic meaning of the tree, which appears in many cultures, is "as the center of the world, a living axis topping the summit of the world mountain and reaching up to heaven." Eliot, *Myths,* 110.

2. The tree is "a symbol of man, or the human being on all planes, as a replica in small, of the Divine being in whose image man is made. As God is a Tree of Life, so man is the same. . . .

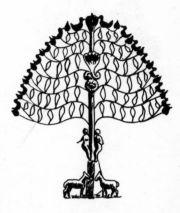

The 'Tree' is indeed the best analogue that could be given for the 'Kingdom' as above and so below. For, as a diagram of the evolution of the Divine Life, the growth from the seed, the sprout, roots, trunk, branches, leaves, flower and fruit, typify the entire cosmic process, and serve to show how gloriously and wonderfully the Great Spiritual Universe, the archetype of the phenomenal cosmos, is contrived, energised, and sustained by the Master Builder—its Source and Centre." Gaskell, *Dictionary of All Scriptures and Myths,* 765, 766.

3. "The legends concerning the tree of the golden apples or figs, which yields honey or ambrosia, guarded by dragons, in which the life, the fortune, the glory, the strength, and the riches of the hero have their beginning, are numerous among every people of Aryan origin, in India, and in Persia, in Russia and in Poland, in Sweden and in Germany, in Greece and in Italy." Gubernatis, *Zoological Mythology,* II, 410.

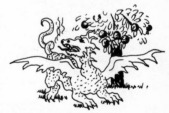

The spiritual individual "is like a tree planted by streams of water, that yields its fruit in its season and its leaf does not wither." *The Holy Bible,* Psalms 1:3.

"The kingdom of Heaven is like a grain of mustard seed which a man took and sowed in his field; it is the smallest of all seeds but when it has grown it is the greatest of shrubs and becomes a tree, so that the birds of the air come and make nests in its branches." *The Holy Bible,* Matthew 13:31.

vrikshasana

TREE

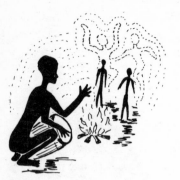

4. Freund, *Myths of Creation,* 108-109.

   The tree has been used in myths of many cultures to explain the origin of the human race. See *Encyclopedia of World Mythology* for further examples.

5. In a tale of the Asmats, a tribe in Dutch New Guinea, a lonely magician yearned for companionship, so he carved some wooden figures and brought them to life by beating rhythmically on a drum. Freund, *Myths of Creation,* 107.

6. Tree worship was widespread in Europe. According to James Frazer this was a natural occurrence because of the "immense primaeval forests, in which the scattered clearings must have appeared like islets in an ocean of green." Frazer, *The Golden Bough,* 144.

   The Druids, Mayans, and Israelis all performed their rites within sacred groves of trees. It is interesting to see the similarity of religious practices among widely diverse cultures. See Churchward, *Signs and Symbols of Primordial Man,* 181.

7. Campbell, *Primitive Mythology,* 212. According to Campbell, this same tree is found in the higher civilizations of the Maya-Aztec and Peruvian late periods as well as in Egypt, Mesopotamia, India, and China.

8. "In Buddhist legend . . . the whole sense of the teaching is that one should penetrate that guarded gate and discover that tree— the Bodhi Tree, the tree of the 'Waking to Omniscience.'" Campbell, *The Mythic Image,* 194.

9. Peck, *Egyptian Drawings,* 112.

10. *Larousse World Mythology,* 365.

11. Ibid., 399.

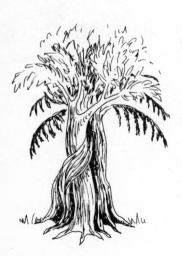

12. "Medieval Christians had many legends about the olive. One of the basic . . . ones was that when Adam died the angel guarding the garden of Eden . . . gave Seth a seed each of olive, cedar and cypress. These were placed in Adam's mouth and eventually sprouted from his grave, forming a single triple-trunked tree. It was from this tree that Noah's dove plucked the

symbolic leaf, beneath this tree that David wept, and it was this tree that Solomon cut down. Too hard to be formed into timber, it was used as a bridge on which the Queen of Sheba crossed a bog. Eventually it formed the basis of the Cross." *Encyclopedia of World Mythology*, 244.

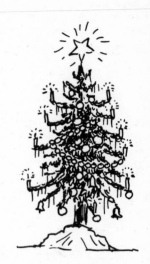

13. "There seems at one time to have been a widely spread notion that the Cross of Christianity was a *Tree*. It was not until A.D. 608 that Christ was represented as a man on a cross." Bayley, *The Lost Language of Symbolism*, part 2, 267.

14. "The evergreen tree is the Winter Solstice; the New Year and a fresh beginning. It is the tree of rebirth and immortality, the Tree of Paradise of lights and gifts, shining by night. Each light is a soul and the lights also represent the sun, moon and stars shining in the branches of the Cosmic Tree." Cooper, *Illustrated Encyclopaedia of Traditional Symbols*, 35.

15. A *samana* is an ascetic.

16. *Questions of King Milinda*, VII, 6, 9.

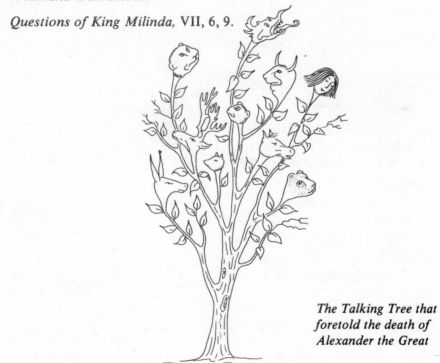

The Talking Tree that foretold the death of Alexander the Great

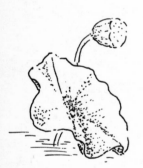

Padma means
"lotus."In this posture
the legs are crossed,
the feet resting on the
thighs with the soles
facing up. The spine
is erect, the hands
either placed on the
knees, palms up, or
resting in the lap.

padmasana
LOTUS

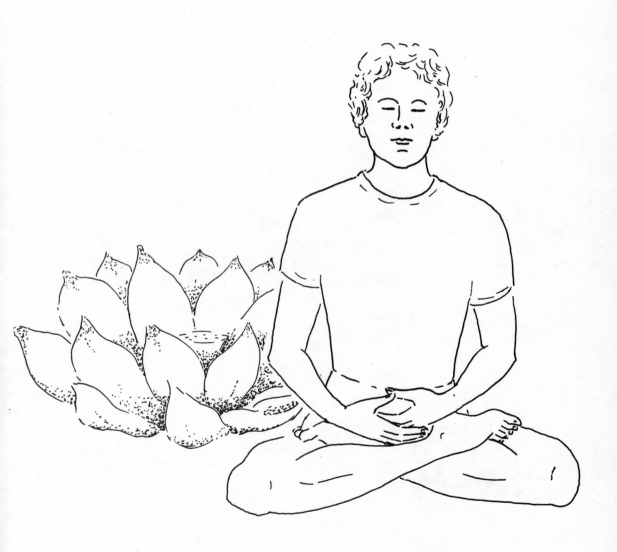

"The lotus grows in muddy waters but this flower does not show any trace of it; so we have to live in the world."

B.K.S. Iyengar

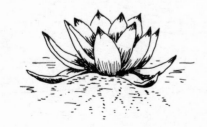

padmasana
LOTUS

THE FLOWERS OF BOTH the water lily and the lotus are associated with exceptional beauty but, because they float on the surface of the water, they are not easily within reach. Their roots are in the mud and they grow up through the muddy water. Likewise, the waters of selfishness are muddy and slippery, and the flowering of Consciousness in the aspirant sometimes seems impossible to attain.

Not only the flower of the lotus, but the posture itself, appears so glamorous that its achievement seems worthwhile, regardless of its difficulty. It is called the "royal posture" and one who can do Padmasana with ease is fortunate. It is as if one assumes, with the lotus posture, the beauty, the grace, and the divinity of the flower.

The lotus symbolizes the opposites of birth and death, male and female, and the interaction of the creative forces. It has generally been considered the "Flower of Light" and has appeared with the sun gods of the Egyptians and Hindus, with Semitic moon gods, and with the Great Mother as lunar goddess.[1] The veneration of the lotus is probably best illustrated in the variety of its display in houses, temples, and churches. In Europe, where the lotus does not grow naturally, its sacredness was symbolized by the rose in the stained glass windows, called "rose windows," of the old cathedrals and churches. Beautiful mosaic domes, or even ceilings, also are to be found in the design of the lotus in Italy and Spain—in fact, in almost any Mediterranean country.

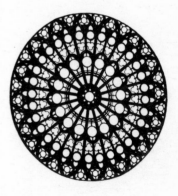

To the Chinese the lotus "represents past, present and future, since the plant bears buds, flowers and fruit at the same time."[2] Its value can also be seen in the daily life of the people, who use all parts of the plant.[3] The lotus is shown as the single most important flower in Egyptian monuments and paintings

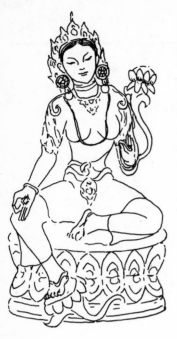

because of its use in religious rites of ancient times.[4] The blue lotus is the special flower of Tara, the Mother of Compassion for Tibetan Buddhists. Wherever the lotus flower has made its home, it has immediately created an atmosphere of sacredness, beauty, and awe.

The body must be trained to achieve the lotus posture. In spite of the subtleness of the psychology of this pose, it is not without its strong effects on body and mind. In this traditional meditation posture, there comes a stillness—first without, then within. Allow these thoughts about the lotus to float in your mind.

PADMASANA: Lotus Posture

Beauty, floating, not easily within reach, selfishness, muddy and slippery, difficult, royal posture, grace, divinity, birth and death, male and female, creative forces, Flower of Light, buds, flowers and fruit, sacredness, beauty, awe, trained, subtle psychology, strong effects, stillness

In the East the lotus represents levels of consciousness, and the fully open flower is associated with the Buddha, as well as with most other important religious figures and deities. It is indicative of a throne of a very special preciousness. Lord Buddha, who is considered "lotus born," and the World Mother in her many names (108 names in all), are shown seated or standing on a lotus, which presents them to us as being beyond human nature.[5] For both Hindus and Buddhists the lotus is symbolic of spiritual attainment, the flowering of human potential.

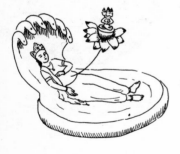

One of the most charming stories among the many that speak of the creation of the universe, describes the center of the lotus as the cradle of the world, and the stem of the lotus as rooted in the navel of Vishnu. The essence (Brahma) of life originated from this place. Each one of the petals symbolizes a particular world, as well as a stage in an aspirant's development.

The earth is sometimes compared to a lotus leaf floating on the surface of the cosmic waters.[6] Frequently the physical body is called the earth, providing the conditions in which consciousness can grow; the light of both, we are assured, is the same. The innate nature of the human being is divine, and the shining lotus of the inner spiritual being will appear in all its glory when the dirty waters have receded and the mud has been wiped off.

There is another peculiarity about the lotus which sets it apart; a drop of water on a lotus leaf has a silvery shine, reflecting the green of the leaf from below and the blue of the sky above.

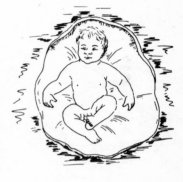

The perfect roundness of the green leaves, with their tiny rims, brings to mind tales of babies who were found lying, well-protected, on those leaves that are strong enough to carry the weight of an infant. Could it be that at some time unwanted babies were exposed in this way, to be discovered by compassionate souls? Was this the origin of the idea that a great soul was projected into the world, or "lotus born"?

Perhaps the lotus leaf could be thought of as the cradle for the new birth of the spiritual baby within us, in the lotus pond of the mind.

PADMASANA: Lotus Posture

Levels of consciousness, Buddha, spiritual attainment, flowering of human potential, manifestation, shining lotus, dirty waters, drop of water, silvery shine, reflecting, perfect roundness, cradle, new birth, spiritual baby

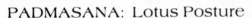

The large leaves of the lotus are also a protection for small fish. As the plant moves with the water, offering no resistance, the waves from the swift movements of the fish create a dance in unison with everything that floats on the surface. To be entangled among the stems of the lotus and its many leaves is no easy matter for a swimmer. It is almost as if the lotus wants to hold on to anything that comes into its midst, so that it can

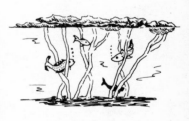

padmasana

LOTUS

become as beautiful and light and gently-dancing as the flowers themselves. The beauty of the lotus and the murkiness of the water point to the opposites that make up life.

We are reminded of *The Odyssey of Homer* in which Odysseus and his men were blown off course and ended up in the Land of the Lotus Eaters. When the men were given the "honey-sweet fruit of the lotus" to eat, they forgot their duties and their way home, wanting only to stay with the lotus-eating people, feeding on the lotus. When human beings come into contact with the beauties of spiritual life they want to remain there, and not return to their former murky lives.

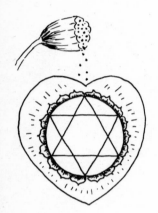

It is fascinating to learn about the longevity of the seeds of this plant. Botanists recently found a lotus seed that had remained dormant for 2,000 years, and that sprouted after it was placed in water. Similarly, the spiritual seed, which is within the heart of everyone—made up of love, consideration, beauty, peace, and happiness—will come to life given the right circumstances, even after being dormant for uncounted births. It is that spiritual essence that conveys the idea of eternal life. It is from the center of the lotus within that the Light emanates.[7]

The flower of the lotus or water lily has a protective layer of green leaves that unfurl slowly, giving at first only a glimpse of the bud, and its color, underneath. The aspirant, nourishing those spiritual qualities, often needs a protective environment until the flower is grown enough to withstand the storms. It is only through the pursuit of Divine Wisdom that one can, like the lotus flower, keep one's head above the surface of the turbulent waters of life.[8]

REFLECTIONS: Lotus

The lotus does not grow in crystal clear streams, but in the collected debris that has sunk to the bottom of the lake. Yet, as the flower slowly emerges through the muddy waters, it is not stained. Occasionally it does happen that a lotus opens its blossom just below the surface of the water, prematurely. Similarly, it is possible for an aspirant to have spiritual experiences before clearing the muddy waters of the mind; but eventually the flower of Consciousness will emerge, pure and unstained.

The true aspirant is not stained by the muddy waters of surrounding life. Spiritual awareness will increase by continually seeking to eradicate the selfish expressions of the lower nature. It is in that control of body and mind that the term *science of Yoga* is most applicable. Seek no comfort when the face is wet from tears. The pain of tearing away from needs, desires, and self-created worlds is deep. In the early stages a feeling of sentimentality will make the sacrifice appear to be great because one really doesn't want to give up that which creates the pain. But Liberation is closer when this work on self can be a gift from the heart.

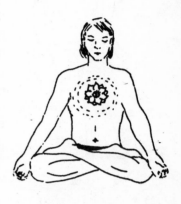

The conquest of self is an arduous one. But we cannot expect Liberation to come to us as a gift from God or the Guru, without our own effort. The disappointment that this is so may be projected on to the teacher; but criticism of others will not remove the flaws. When a high degree of spiritual awareness has been achieved, the inner being will appear to the aspirant, like the flower of the lotus, unsullied by any mud-slinging. Let this be the resolve, or the renunciation, of the aspirant: to remember to focus on faith, thereby recognizing that faith is a power in itself.

The sage Nagasena, having stated that the lotus remains untainted, continues to explain that water, whenever it falls on the lotus leaf, simply rolls off. Once an aspirant has attained the power of meditation and faith, the temptations of lust, anger, cruelty, and many other types of negative thoughts, will also flow off and disperse; they will not attach themselves, because pride, self-righteousness, and self-will are scattered away. The aspirant is born in a world as muddy as the waters in which the lotus is born, but the flower of spirituality is

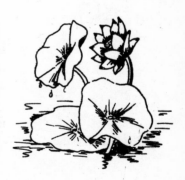

padmasana

LOTUS

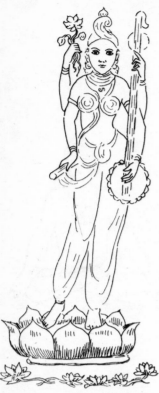

Saraswati, Devi of Speech

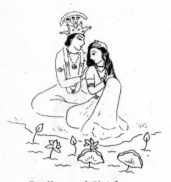

Radha and Krishna

untainted. Even fame, honor, and veneration cannot attach themselves. When the wind blows over the water, it makes ripples, and even the lotus may tremble. If awareness is directed toward the discovery of the Light, then the lotus may be shaken in the storm but it will not be destroyed.

In the *Satapatha Brahmana,* the lotus is described as having a very important place in consecration ceremonies, a lotus flower being presented each time oblations are offered; for example, Saraswati, the Devi of Speech, is given a lotus flower along with an oblation of rice. The lotus confirms the sacredness of an offering and, for the aspirant, can be symbolic for the dedication to the Most High.

The *Gitagovinda* of Jayadeva stresses the significance of the lotus in erotic love. Padmini is the lotus-lady, concocting potions and perfumes to attract a lover. According to Lee Siegel's commentary on this book,

> the lotus-image has a dynamic ambiguity, a tensive quality, as a symbol—it suggests the erotic and the religious and as such draws the two dimensions closely together, holds them sensuously together. When Radha suffers with thoughts of lotuses the suggestion is conventionally erotic—lotuses suggest and enhance the erotic mood and hence cause the separated lover to grieve; but as the lotus, with its religious overtones, is also an emblem of Krsna as the Lord the suggestion is also devotional. . . . Human loving, through the symbol, is identified with the vast energy at work in the creation of the universe.[9]

The lotus and the water lily will open only after a minimum of four hours of sunlight. From this the aspirant can learn that the inner lotus needs the light of the Divine Wisdom, nourished by devotion, in order to experience renunciation as a happy deliverance, rather than an arduous task.

When the effort required to sit in Padmasana with ease is understood as symbolic for the stilling of the monkey-mind so the Light of the lotus within can shine forth, it will be seen to be indeed worthwhile. Remaining clear-eyed, beyond the clouds of emotion, the reward of the experience emerging in the center of the heart lotus will be a taste of bliss never before known.

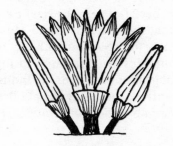

Egyptian lotus

1. According to Heinrich Zimmer, the goddess who stands or is seated on a lotus dates back to ancient societies that worshipped Mother Earth in many parts of the world. Images of this goddess have been found in the Near East, in lands around the Mediterranean, the Black Sea, and Mesopotamia. "Thus, she furnishes a clew to pre-Aryan linkages between India and the sources of our Western Tradition of myth and symbol." When patriarchal groups took over the Indus Civilization they took the goddess off the lotus seat and put Brahma in her place. Zimmer, *Myths and Symbols in Indian Art and Civilization,* 92, 96.

2. Cooper, *Illustrated Encyclopaedia of Traditional Symbols,* 101.

3. See C. A. S. Williams, *Outlines of Chinese Symbolism and Art Motives,* for a description of the practical uses of the lotus among the Chinese.

4. Nefer-Tem is sometimes represented as holding in his hands the lotus scepter surmounted by plumes. "Sometimes he appears in religious scenes with the lotus flower, or the lotus flower and plumes upon his head." In the Pyramid Text of Unas "the dead king is compared to a lotus at the nostrils of the great Sekhem. . . . 'Unas hath risen like Nefer-Tem from the lotus to the nostrils of Ra.'" Budge, *Gods of the Egyptians,* vol. 1, 520-521.

5. "The lotus flower, by reproducing from its own matrix, rather than in the soil, is a symbol of spontaneous generation. And the lotus which serves as seat or throne for the Buddha indicates, therefore, divine birth. . . . The blossom of the lotus offered by the worshipper to the divinity signifies the surrender of his own existence to its origin, the abandonment of his own nature to the Buddha, the renouncement of an independent existence." Saunders, *Mudra,* 159.

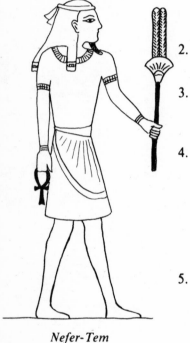

Nefer-Tem

padmasana

LOTUS

6. "The lotus signifies ontologically a solid base in the middle of the possibilities of existence, a birth and a manifestation which are produced essentially in the intelligible world and later also in the world of the senses; it signifies ethically the detachment particular to him who is in the world but who is not attached to it." Ibid., 160.

7. The *Chandogya Upanishad* (8:1.1) speaks of the nature of the soul: "Now, what is here in this city of Brahma, is an abode, a small lotus-flower (the heart). Within that is a small space. What is within that, should be searched out; that, assuredly, is what one should desire to understand." Hume, *Thirteen Principle Upanishads*, 262.

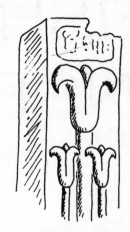

Egyptian lotus column

Similarly, in the *Maitri Upanishad* (6:2): "Now, he who dwells within the lotus of the heart and eats food is the same as that solar fire which dwells in the sky, called Time, the invisible, which eats all things as his food. What is the lotus and of what does it consist? This lotus, assuredly, is the same as space. These four quarters of heaven and the four intermediate quarters are the form of its leaves. These two, the breathing spirit and the sun, go forth toward each other." Ibid., 424.

8. Like the lotus, everyone is exposed to water. Water will change and adapt quickly to the movement of the air, to different temperatures, to its confinement, to deep currents, or to waves on the surface. It offers a stimulus for comparison with life itself; for example, "getting into hot water" refers to a risky, difficult situation that could be very unpleasant. The unpleasantness of getting one's feet into cold water refers to a different type of problem. Think also of the meaning of such phrases as "not making any waves," "not stirring things up," or "riding the crest of the wave."

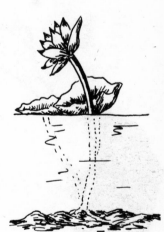

The lotus, with its long flexible stem, can ride any waves that the wind may whip up. As the depth of the water determines the length of the stem, the flexibility, yet firmness, of mind and body are interlocking.

9. Siegel, *Sacred and Profane Dimensions of Love,* 197-198.

LOTUS

FISH·REPTILES·
INSECTS

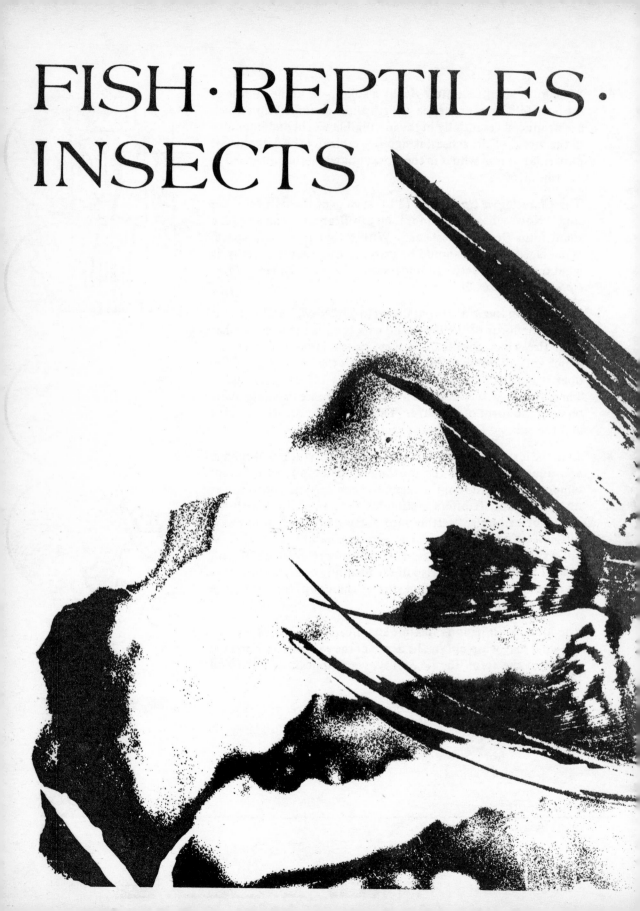

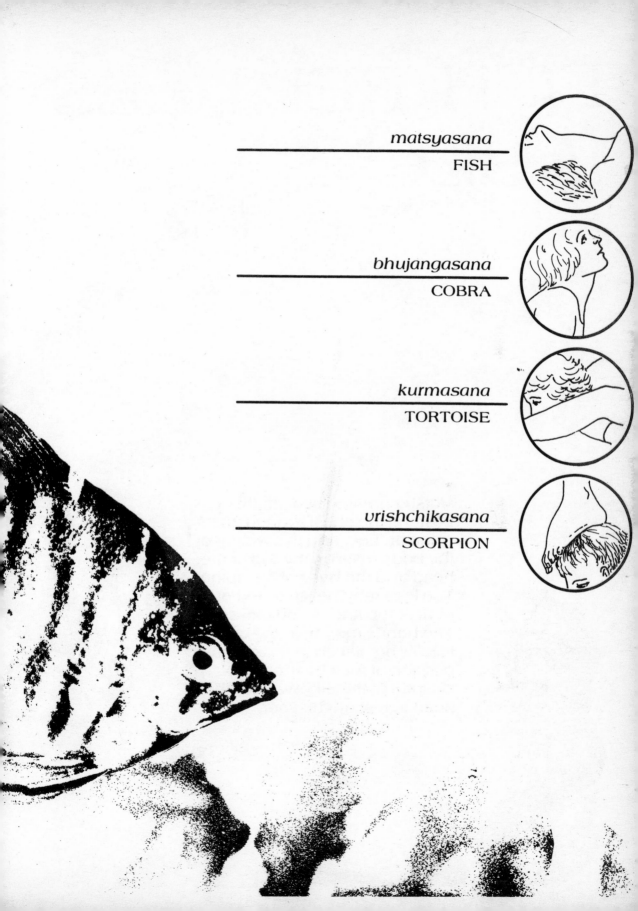

matsyasana
FISH

bhujangasana
COBRA

kurmasana
TORTOISE

vrishchikasana
SCORPION

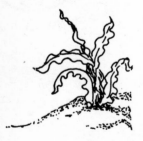

Matsya means "fish." In this posture, the chest is open, the spine arched, and the weight of the body rests on the top of the head and the base of the spine. The legs may be stretched out or bent at the knees and crossed. The hands may hold the crossed feet, or be placed in the namaste position at the chest, or be clasped at the elbows over the head to rest on the floor.

matsyasana

FISH

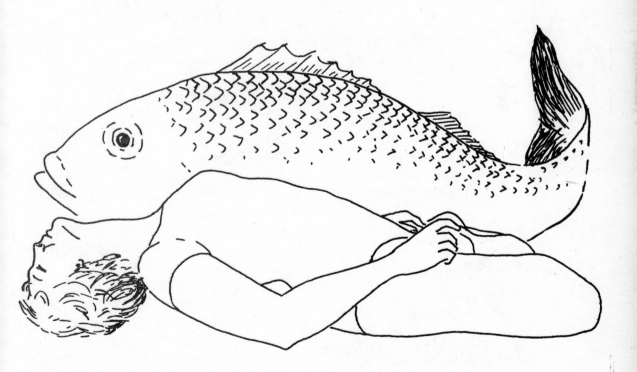

"When the chest is opening, the mind is opening, and we feel emotionally shiny, and stability comes. This is emotional stability."

B.K.S. Iyengar

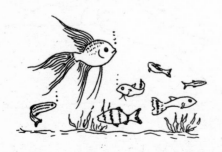

matsyasana

FISH

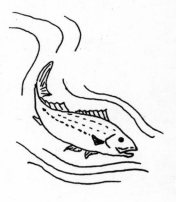

Water[1] HAS A FORMIDABLE power, demanding that the body of the fish that lives in it be streamlined.[2] Water is a resistant element, as one discovers when rowing a boat. For the fish to "part the waters," requires strength and flexibility of the spine. Fish have fins and tails that are strong, yet at the same time delicate, which lends grace and elegance to their motions. They can move swiftly or remain almost motionless; their agility is their protection in a hostile environment in which the bigger eats the smaller.

Watching fish swim in water, one becomes aware of their constant restless movements as they seek food for nourishment. People also seek nourishment, primarily of an emotional type until they begin to understand, through the practice of the asana, that unconsciously they may really be seeking spiritual nourishment.

In this posture as you lift up the chest, causing the back to curve, you will have many passing thoughts such as, What am I lifting up—my lungs, my heart? Why that strain on my throat, my neck? Am I stiff-necked? Do I have rigid concepts? an unbending will? In Matsyasana the chest—and the heart—are exposed. They are the highest points of the body, like the top of a small mountain. Strength becomes recognizable when one can relax in this posture in spite of its vulnerability; an underlying faith and trust may now be directly experienced.

MATSYASANA: Fish Posture

Power, streamlined, resistant, flexibility, grace, elegance, delicate, swift, motionless, agility, restless, nourishment, chest and heart, stiff-necked, rigid, unbending will, vulnerability, faith, trust

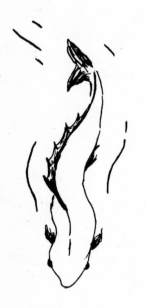

The fish lives in an element in which many other creatures have their lives, too. Not every one is dangerous, but not every one is friendly, either. Human beings can live on the surface of the earth—in the lowlands or on top of mountains—and also for short periods in water. Everywhere they meet with their own kind or other species with whom they have to share the space.

To be flexible like the fish does not mean to be spineless. Fish have light and delicate spines which, supported by their muscles, give them a strength from which the practitioner of asanas can learn a great deal. An inflexible spine gives a person the appearance of age. Problems in this area point to a poor self-image, depression, aggressiveness, or a strength of self-will that prevents flexibility, a very important factor in human relations. Gurus I have met have demonstrated this flexibility by being as hard as steel with one disciple and as soft as butter with another.

The sense perceptions of fish are somewhat different from those of humans. Fish, like human beings, are sensitive to touch and taste, but ichthyologists have found that they also have a sixth sense[3] that enables them to cope in their unique world. They have no ears and this gives them an extraordinary sensitivity to the vibration of sound.

This sixth sense may be the source of the myths, fables, and stories that abound regarding the fish.[4] The fish produces a paradox in the human mind, not only because it is such an ancient symbol, but because it exercises great personal power and influence for individuals. To speak of mystical qualities is not to deny the historical aspects; they have indeed more often than not preceded the myth.

In Hindu legends we have, among others of importance, the story of the great sage Vyasa who was born of a fish virgin.[5] The Greeks said the fish carries the human soul in its belly;[6] should the significance of this legend be sought in the time when fish were eaten only by the priests as sacramental food?

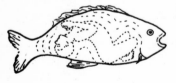

The Tibetans have two fish facing each other on a lotus pedestal as a symbol for happiness. And in the *Egyptian Book of the Dead* two fish are believed to swim beside the boat of the sun god to protect it from evil.

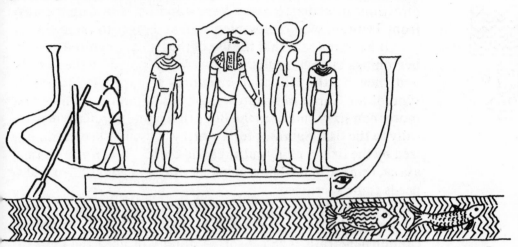

This incredible human mind also gave birth to the great god of the Sumerians, E-A (Oannes), believed to be half-man and half-fish. From the minds of the Mesopotamians emerged a woman with a fishtail, who dwelt in the southern oceans, its tides and waves governed by her heartbeat. The Sumerians called their mermaid NIN-MAH. The Virgin Mary's name in Hebrew is Miriam, which means "brine of the sea"; more poetically expressed, it could also mean "essence" or "heart of the sea."

The present-day interest in astrology seems to be a revival of an ancient science. The study of the heavens moved the people of ancient times to worship the gods that they believed inhabited the heavenly bodies. For instance, Indian astrology is based on the avatar, Vishnu, who incarnated as a great fish to save the world and to preserve life and the Vedas.[7] George Michanowsky speaks also of the Vela star god, E-A, saying

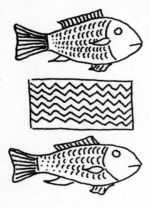

that one of his names had been HA-AN, meaning "fish of heaven." The constellation of Pisces is not the two fish swimming in opposite directions as seen in modern astrology; in the old tradition, the fish were thought of as swimming in the same direction, in order to carry Venus and her son Cupid away from Typhon, who represented a great danger to them.

It has been said that the use of the fish as a symbol had its beginnings in pagan cults. Later it was adopted by the Jewish and then by the Christian religions. It appears often as a symbol for Christ in scriptures, art, and literature. There are more than sixty entries in the Bible that name or refer symbolically to the fish. Sacrifice for a worthy cause has been symbolized by the fish in many cultures and creeds. When you do this asana, think about what is being sacrificed in your life, or what needs to be sacrificed.

The mind, like a fish, searches the depths of the unconscious, the dark and murky waters where the light from above cannot penetrate. The censoring mind will need the light of insights that come from the heart, from the open chest in this asana, to obtain a full vision. It is the ambiguous mind that looks everywhere in order to escape from true insights, searching to find elusive treasures it can own.

It is important for the aspirant to discriminate between being truly sensitive and being touchy or easily hurt. Most people are sensitive only to their own egos. Water itself represents the unconscious and emotions—tears of sorrow or joy—in schools of Western psychology. In the Kundalini system water is the controlling element of the second chakra (Svadisthana) and stands for imagination, while the third (Manipura) represents emotions. Combined, these two powers make humans most vulnerable—gulping, sinking, dying, or being elevated, strengthened in faith, resurrected from the depths of despair. When the aspirant can swim with ease in the waters of imagination and emotions, the sixth sense—an awareness and concern for others—will develop.

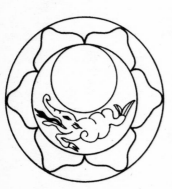

The second chakra

matsyasana

FISH

MATSYASANA: Fish Posture

Dangerous, friendly, own kind, other species,
share the space, spineless, strength, age,
youthful, poor self-image, depression,
aggressiveness, self-will, human relations,
sensitive, sixth sense, vibration, sacrifice,
unconscious, light, insights, censoring mind,
ambiguous mind, escape, treasures, touchy,
imagination, emotions, gulping, sinking,
dying, elevated, faith, resurrected, despair,
awareness, concern

The story of a great flood on earth has made its appearance in many cultures and religions, and therefore it is not surprising to find it in Indian texts. Vishnu, in his aspect of the preserver, was concerned about the continuance of the human race. He came to Manu, father of mankind, in the form of a very small fish, asking that he be cared for until he grew large enough to swim in the ocean. In return he promised Manu to save him from the flood that would destroy the earth, and he ordered Manu to make ready a sea-going craft large enough so that a pair from each species of creature could board. When the flood came, Manu attached the boat to the horn of the fish and with it sailed away to the northern mountain.

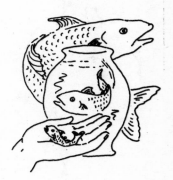

The body is the earth and the emotions are the waters that flood the mind, preventing clear sight. How much can anybody "see" when flooded with emotions? Suddenly the mind is recognized to be not only simplistic and ambiguous, but also literal and censoring. It becomes essential to cut through the waters of emotions in order to see clearly. The pursuit of awareness brings about clarity of mind. The vigilance of practice aimed at knowing oneself will reveal the two selves, the conscious and unconscious. Manu survived the flood, and the aspirant can survive the turbulence of life by being sensitive to and following divine guidance.

Do only the faithful swim with ease, like the fish, in the waters of life?

FISH

REFLECTIONS: Fish

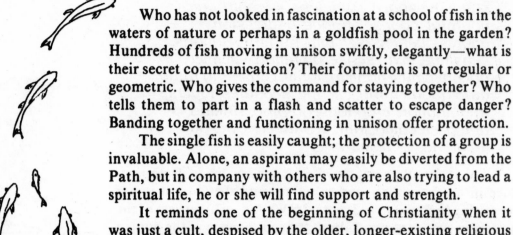

Who has not looked in fascination at a school of fish in the waters of nature or perhaps in a goldfish pool in the garden? Hundreds of fish moving in unison swiftly, elegantly—what is their secret communication? Their formation is not regular or geometric. Who gives the command for staying together? Who tells them to part in a flash and scatter to escape danger? Banding together and functioning in unison offer protection.

The single fish is easily caught; the protection of a group is invaluable. Alone, an aspirant may easily be diverted from the Path, but in company with others who are also trying to lead a spiritual life, he or she will find support and strength.

It reminds one of the beginning of Christianity when it was just a cult, despised by the older, longer-existing religious societies. The members of the cult would draw a fish in the sand as a sign by which to recognize each other. It was a passmark when they secretly congregated together to give strength and support to each other. The "way of the fish" was adopted without a particular structure or design, but all branches and members were united in a common goal and in their commitment to that goal.

Down through the ages the element of water has had a strong appeal in many forms: wishing wells, springs of pure water from the rocks—creating promises of eternal youth, Divine Wisdom, and many other powers. Humans everywhere have also been fascinated with the reflection of themselves on the quiet surface of water. The aspirant needs to spend time in reflection, gazing deeply into the pool of the mind.

Did this fascination with water stem from thought associations about the beginning of human life when the embryo rides weightlessly in the salty amniotic sac, like the fish in the sea? Fingers and toes are webbed like fish fins, the eyes are wide open, with no eyelids—resembling the fish—before the next stage of development into a fetus. This has led some scientists to believe that human evolution started in the salty waters of the ocean.

Human fascination with the water, with exploring the vastness and the depth of the sea and the many forms of life in it, has accounted for a number of incredible stories. Reports about the intelligence of the porpoise or the killer whale have contributed to keeping alive human imagination. Many of the stories about sea monsters and mermaids (an especially moving example, being half-human and half-fish) were like seeds sprouting colorfully in the minds of seafarers or islanders surrounded by the sea.

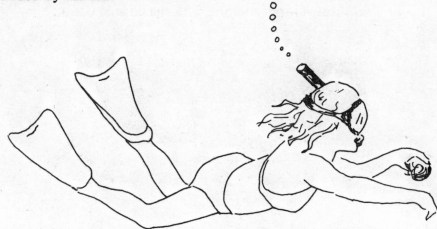

The sea within us harbors many creatures of our imagination—frightening monsters and beautiful mermaids, afraid of each other's strength. They are wonderful symbols for the ongoing struggle. Their impact, were they to surface, would be as astounding as seeing an actual sea monster or mermaid.

The flow in the unconscious is like an undercurrent in the great water. To survive in that unknown territory it is necessary to move slowly, carefully, watchfully, with the right motivation, from a position of strength and flexibility. Stubborn resistance blocks the flow. To allow the heart to expand gives release and a deep feeling of relief when the posture is finally

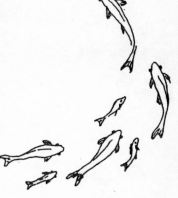

matsyasana

FISH

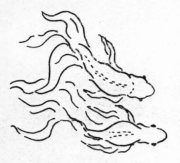

completed. Learning to live more in the unconscious, opening up those areas that, like the sea, may once have been our habitat, helps the unfathomable depths within to lose their threat.

The Light of the heart can now illumine the mind. The Self is freed, if only for a moment, to rise high in the stillness that allows devotional feelings to flower; and the perfume of gratitude can envelop the entire being, thus bringing on itself a wonderful blessing. Like a fish in the sea, the aspirant can learn to swim freely in the ocean of Divine Wisdom. To strive for it means one is not yet part of it. The little drop of consciousness longs to unite with the cosmic ocean.

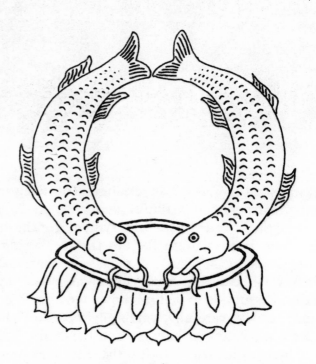

*Two fish facing each other on a lotus pedestal:
the Tibetan symbol for happiness*

matsyasana

FISH

REFERENCE NOTES: Fish

1. Water is one of four elements that are among the eight support-ing and illuminating powers of all beings. The others are: earth, air, fire, speech, mind, sight, and hearing. *Prasna Upanishad*, 2:2. The *Bhagavad Gita*, 7:4, names eight natures: earth, water, fire, air, ether, mind, intellect, and egoism.

   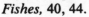

   In the Kundalini system, each chakra, or level of awareness, is associated with an element: the first contains the quality earth; the second, water; the third, fire; the fourth, air; and the fifth, ether. See Swami Sivananda Radha, *Kundalini: Yoga for the West*.

2. Ommanney, *The Fishes,* 36, 37.

   For the power of water from the yogic point-of-view, see Swami Sivananda Radha, *Kundalini: Yoga for the West*, 115.

3. Fish have "a true sixth sense which makes them acutely aware of very subtle changes in the flow of water around them. This 6th sense is unique to them and it operates by means of nerve organs located in a canal system underneath the skin." This canal system "can be seen on the side of the fish as a file of scales shaped differently from the others." Ommanney, *The Fishes,* 40, 44.

   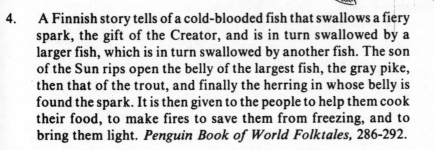

4. A Finnish story tells of a cold-blooded fish that swallows a fiery spark, the gift of the Creator, and is in turn swallowed by a larger fish, which is in turn swallowed by another fish. The son of the Sun rips open the belly of the largest fish, the gray pike, then that of the trout, and finally the herring in whose belly is found the spark. It is then given to the people to help them cook their food, to make fires to save them from freezing, and to bring them light. *Penguin Book of World Folktales,* 286-292.

5. A fish, who was really a nymph under enchantment, swallowed the seed of King Vasu and in ten months was caught by a fisherman who discovered a boy and a beautiful girl in the fish's belly. The boy was adopted by the king but the girl, named Satyavati (Truth), remained as the fisherman's daughter because she had a fishy smell. Seduced by a yogi who was overcome by her beauty, she pleaded with him not to violate her purity. The yogi, impressed by her character, granted her wish to have a sweet smell and, after she gave birth to a boy, restored her virginity. The boy's name was Vyasa, who helped to interpret the Vedas and was author of some of the Puranas. Campbell, *The Masks of God: Oriental Mythology,* 328-330, 336.

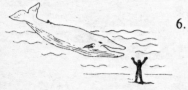

6. In the Jewish tradition, Jonah is spoken of as having been "reborn from the whale . . . of whom it is said in the *Midrash* that in the belly of the fish he typifies the soul of man swallowed by Sheol." Campbell, *The Masks of God: Creative Mythology*, 13.

7. This is a popular Hindu myth about a time when the human mind was so highly developed that written language was not necessary. The Vedas had been preserved by being committed to memory; so if man had died, the wisdom would have been lost.

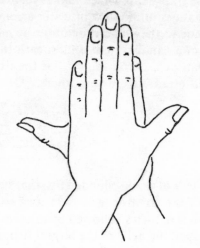

Matsya Mudra: East Indian prayer dance mudra *(symbolic hand gestures) representing* matsya *(the fish)*

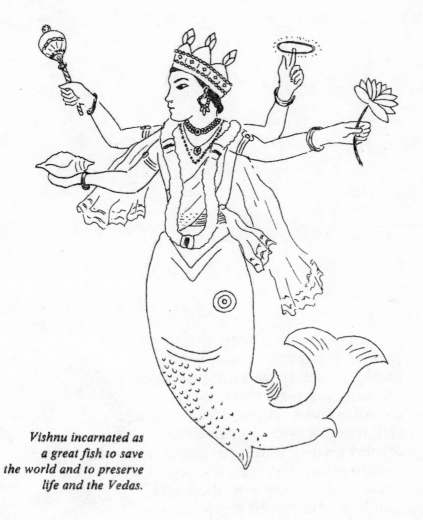

*Vishnu incarnated as
a great fish to save
the world and to preserve
life and the Vedas.*

matsyasana •*145*

FISH

Bhujanga means "serpent." The pose starts from a downward-facing position with the palms of the hands flat on the floor below the shoulders. The spine is lengthened and the buttocks firmed as the head and chest are slowly lifted. The elbows stay close to the body and the eyes look up. The return to the original position is made slowly.

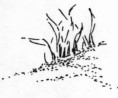

bhujangasana
COBRA

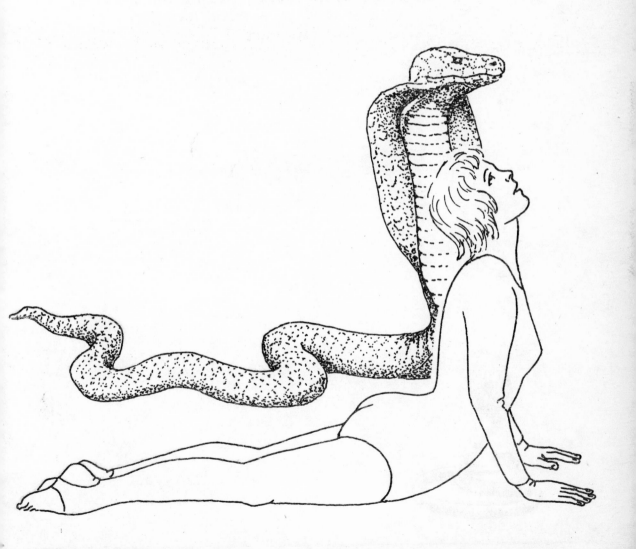

"Like a snake, the spine should be moved from end to end; when the head moves, the movement is transmitted to the tail."
                                    B.K.S. Iyengar

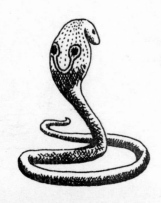

bhujangasana

COBRA

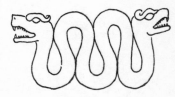

THERE ARE VERY FEW people who are not afraid of snakes. The most powerful and fearsome is the cobra. It is feared even among people such as the Eskimos, who live where there are no snakes. My research shows that the symbol of the cobra can be found in twenty-two of the major countries of the world. Its deadly poison means instant death, yet its ability to shed its skin symbolizes renewal and resurrection.[1] It represents fertility,[2] birth and death; wisdom and temptation; good and evil; the paradox of the struggle of life.

The psychological implication of snakes lies in the fear of being over-powered unexpectedly by the poison that life throws at us at every turn—the collapse of economics, of health, of life. The battle is constant. The result is often exhaustion and helplessness until we realize that, as Saint Paul says, we will never be tempted beyond our capacities.

As I lie prone on the ground in this posture, face down, like a crawling creature, by what effort can I dispel sudden temptation? It is a humbling and fearful position—I could be stepped on. Placing my hands firmly on the ground, raising trunk and head upward—movement without the legs feels different. There is a strange feeling in my stomach and it takes a while before the tightness, the lump in my throat, disappears. My head feels heavy, I am stiff-necked and grim-faced, my heart seems to beat in my throat. Will the chest open, offer itself to the Great Serpent—the great creative force?[3] Will the spiritual power, dormant within me, ever awaken? A snake can make rhythmical movements, but in this asana I feel as if I am locked into position. What am I locked into? Can I shed my old skin? How will I renew myself?

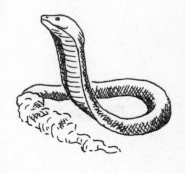

Unaware as I am of any latent potential, the effort needed seems to be enormous. I think of the snake. It has no eyelids; its

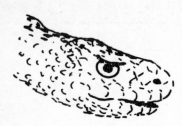

eyes are always open, always seeing, always alert. Will my ignorance stare at me at all times? I cannot stomach this kind of watchfulness. The snake doesn't speak. I scatter many words and thoughts around throughout the day because I don't have the guts to look at what is behind this great silence in myself. Introspection—will it open a can of worms, little snakes too numerous to handle? In my mind's eye, the pictures roll on in painful succession, bringing awareness of their existence but little relief. How can I shed my old skin? Indeed, I want to renew myself.

BHUJANGASANA: Cobra Posture

Powerful, fearsome, deadly poison, sheds its skin, renewal, resurrection, fertility, birth and death, wisdom, temptation, good, evil, paradox, overpowered, exhaustion, helplessness, face down, humbling, stiff-necked, grim-faced, great creative force, rhythmical, locked into position, latent potential, ignorance, watchfulness, introspection, can of worms

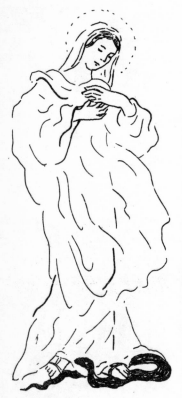

Negative records of the serpent are quite extensive in myths throughout the ages. In the Judeo-Christian tradition the snake is temptation. Man is chased from the Garden of Eden, thereby turning his mind toward procreation to secure the continuation of his kind. But the Virgin Mother is often shown with her foot on the head of a serpent, portraying an idea similar to that of the Hindu god Krishna who dances on the head of the serpent;[4] both signify that awareness can recognize and overcome evil.

In many cultures the snake has been a symbol for the Divine Forces, or the attribute of wisdom. So powerful was the influence of the serpent in the minds of the Norsemen that they engraved it on their swords, and it is prominent in their art. Odin, the supreme god in Norse mythology, occasionally took the form of the serpent, but the highest place was given to the snake as a soul in the "Other World."

The same high place was given to the snake in other countries of Europe and the Middle East. The ornament on Agamemnon's breastplate was made up of three serpents, equated with the rainbow and signifying supreme power above.[5] The Romans had a serpent as an attribute of Minerva, representing wisdom; and the Egyptian god Ra had a snake in his diadem,[6] later copied by many a Pharaoh as it conveyed to the people his wisdom. The two snakes that symbolize Upper and Lower Egypt have their counterpart for the individual in the two selves—the physical-material self and the spiritual self; this illustrates the contradictory nature of this symbol.

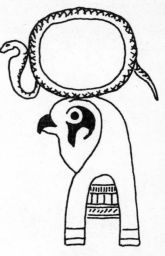

Diadem of Ra

In the large deserts of the Arabian countries tales of serpents and snakes were inspired by people's experiences with them; so serpents could not be excluded from their religious beliefs. In some Arabian tales, the snake is the grateful one. Islam has associated the snake with life and its principles. Ahriman and Angra Mainu are, for the Iranians, the serpents of darkness.

Early history tells us that the Babylonians called the serpent Tiamat, "the footless," "the serpent of darkness," implying chaos and wickedness. The Babylonian E-A, as Lakhmu and Lakhamu, the serpents of the sea, is male and female suggesting that the interaction of masculine and feminine extends to heaven and earth. The idea of rebirth (reincarnation) came also from Babylonia, where the earth-god Ea-En-Ke disseminated to men the knowledge of the world order. Because death was necessary, so was rebirth, if life was to continue.

Man's fear of death led him to nourish a desire for eternal life. The thoughts of death create a sense of horror and themselves become the evil demon. The hour of death being unknown, the demon of death, perhaps in the guise of a deadly snake, seems to hide in the dark to prey noiselessly on its victim. But need the snake be a demon? To the innocent it might appear as a friend. There are many stories in India of events that illustrate this paradox. For instance, cobras, to the

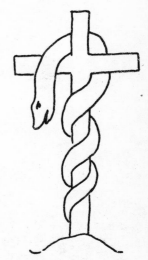

The serpent lifted up

bhujangasana

COBRA

horror of adults who watched, have filled themselves from the milk bowls of little children, not harming them, but treating them as friends.

It seems that some fear is always lurking beneath the surface of life: fear of the sting of criticism, of the poison of depression, the fear of death. Without careful observation, life itself seems to be mystifying and treacherous. When is sex without selfishness, its powerful magnetism pointing to fertility, the instincts rising and striking like a snake? What are the poisons of my mind? Can I watch at all times? My concentration is so poor. Destiny strikes in the moments of life that are most happy and joyful.

The cobra's biological characteristics and habits have contributed a great deal to the development of its symbolism. The structure of some snakes' head and jaws, according to scientists, are designed to allow expansion beyond ordinary limits, which would otherwise be set by the creatures in its surroundings that it must swallow for its survival.

Spiritually speaking, an aspirant's head is also structured for survival in the world. The sensory organs are located here, and the jaws, through their tight clenching, often serve to suppress self-will and anger, or poisonous remarks and cynical judgments. Sometimes it seems that the obstacles are oversized; and yet, as the snake has been structured to handle the obstacles to its survival, so has the aspirant been designed to overcome separation from the divine purpose.

No snake lives alone. There are other related creatures in the environment trying to inject their poison in the struggle of competition for survival. As an aspirant, one will constantly be subjected to poisonous remarks that undermine trust and confidence in oneself, as well as in the Teachings. Adaptation is needed without negating oneself.

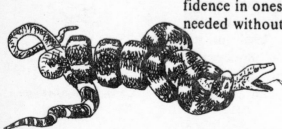

Some cobras are called hooded snakes; they raise their menacing hood for the purpose of increasing fear and submission by bluffing. The most intelligent among all cobras is supposedly the King Cobra. Could this be a link to the snake as a symbol of wisdom?

When the cobra strikes, if the poison enters a large vein, death is very rapid and all so-called antidotes are unavailing. We are told by scientists that some cobras are able to eject a fine stream of poison several feet. In interaction with people, "snakes" may not send their poisonous remarks directly to an aspirant, but casually and under the pretense of non-involvement.

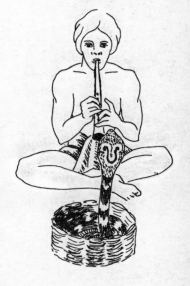

Snake charmers are known mainly in the Eastern countries where travellers have encountered them, their snake "dancing" to the music of the flute.[7] Serpents, being deaf, may react either to the vibration of the sound or to the body movements of the snake charmer. But how do they handle the dangerous creatures? It is said that they become immune by ingesting very small doses of the poisonous venom. This has led to stories which provided a permissible way of referring to sexual intercourse, linking the snake to procreation. "All the story-teller had to do was to transfer the idea from the snake-charmer to a beautiful maiden, and introduce the possibility of passing on a poison thus accumulated. The method of doing this would naturally be intercourse."[8]

It is not only the poison or the venom of a snake that is dangerous; there is also the poison of a glance, the "evil eye." Belief in the evil eye or "fatal look," is widespread in India. The Sanskrit name *drig-visa* or *dristi-visa,* meaning "poison in a glance," goes far back in time. Similar beliefs are found in the Arabian countries. The arrogance in a person's look can be so powerful that it reduces an individual to a helpless victim. We also need to remember Medusa, the Greek Gorgon who, instead of hair, had serpents growing out of her head. Her appearance was so powerful that one glance was sufficient to turn an onlooker into stone.

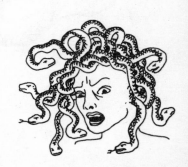

A snake that is a constrictor like the python immobilizes its prey by constricting its body, squeezing out all breath. The aspirant will do well to avoid an atmosphere where spiritual aspirations are stifled. The breath of life is needed not only to keep the body alive, but also as a bridge between two worlds, the tangible and the intangible.

Thoughts such as the following may occur to you as you perform the asana: I want to recoil from the carelessness that has been so long a ruler in my life. The old self is still too forceful. Knowledge is like a rope; I must hold on to it. A little knowledge is like waves—now up, now down. What is the best approach? Why am I so spineless? (The spirit is willing, but the flesh is weak.) Have I made a start? Will I ever penetrate the mystery of life? What is my purpose in life? Wisdom is not penetrating very fast. My heart is not pure. It is filled with lots of other stuff. What stuff? Desires, and more desires. They are not only stuffed into my heart, but into my head also—fueled by emotions. So many attempts to escape. Moving from the dark hiding place in the rocks to allow the sun of wisdom to penetrate.

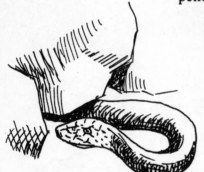

BHUJANGASANA: Cobra Posture

Eternal life, horror, demon, innocent, friend, sting of criticism, poison of depression, magnetism, destiny strikes, competition, poisonous remarks, undermine trust, negating oneself, menacing hood, bluffing, evil eye, helpless victim, constrictors, stifled, recoil from carelessness, knowledge, waves, spineless, desires, fueled by emotions, escape, dark hiding place

What else does a snake mean to me? What can I learn from it? Wisdom does not come running; it glides slowly. Suddenly I am aware of something new, that something has been grasped, learned, has replaced the useless desire of the heart. I am not spineless; my back is growing stronger, ready to ascend from those crevices. A surge of power penetrates my being. I can take a new breath of life. Life is sacred. Life has purpose.

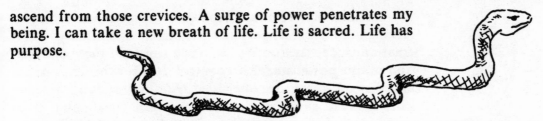

REFLECTIONS: Cobra

Supreme Intelligence dances above the Cosmic ocean where the coiled serpent, Shesha, makes a bed for Vishnu to float on the primordial waters. The seven heads of the serpent are like a protective mantle over the sleeping Vishnu, and the goddess of beauty and wealth, Lakshmi, massages amrita into his feet as a protection against poison. His awakening brings about creation. The water is symbolic for the human seed and the earth for the receptive womb. In this play, creation continues.

The Serpent Ananta (also called Shesha) is the thousand-headed ruler of all serpents, symbolic of the endless, the infinite, of fertility that will go on and on and on. The coils of the serpent are encircling, enticing, coercing humans into being drawn into nature. Those powers of nature—emotions and sex—have to be met and put under the protection of the Divine. The serpent also represents a spiral going upward and another going downward—the nights and days of Brahma, or divine sleep and divine awakening. It is another way of explaining the nights and days of the earth.

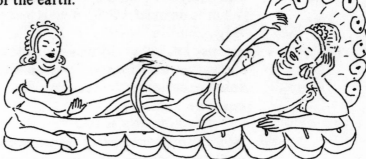

Vishnu on Ananta

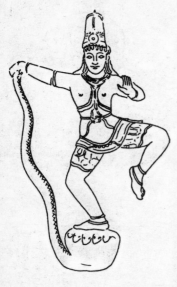

Krishna dances on the head of the serpent Kaliya, representing nature and its power. This sometimes chaotic power is creation in destruction; but Krishna can hold the manifestation of this power under his control. It is for this reason that many of the texts, the *Bhagavad Gita* in particular, refer to Lord Krishna as the single most important focal point. He is the symbol of going beyond nature and its powers, beyond the creative forces that serve only the continuation of the species. When nature stands, like a screen, between the true seeker and the Divine, then focus on Krishna is the only way to go beyond those powerful forces.

Wisdom is a rare characteristic in those whose lives are ruled by uncontrolled emotions. But wisdom is an utter necessity in order to extend life because progress toward enlightenment is so very slow. Snakes move almost noiselessly; wisdom approaches in the same way. But temptation also comes quietly and slowly, suddenly facing us and demanding quick decisions. We become aware at those unexpected moments of the innate wisdom that has always been ours.

Kundalini Shakti symbolizes the serpent power that is ordinarily latent in the human spine.[9] What an incredible promise of the Cosmic Forces, to provide a tool that one can learn to use to move the spiral upward! Helplessness is not one's destiny; it is rather the ability to tap those inner resources. The sudden appearance of temptation or inspirational wisdom can equally grip one's heart. An ensuing sense of panic can delay for a split second the decision to accept or reject. What to do at such a moment is best expressed in the words of Nagasena. He instructs the king that the serpent progresses by means of its belly—by means of knowledge that is digested "at the gut level." Progress by knowledge always means by personal experiences, experiences that are strung together like beads on a mala.

The king also is told that the serpent did not use drugs (soma drink), or any strong intoxicants, because clear thought and clear vision is not obtained in that way; that would be called the road of unrighteousness. It is through the power of discrimination that the aspirant, like a snake, must avoid confrontation when catching sight of anything that is unrighteous. The time lost by engaging in questionable activity or interaction is gone forever. Even a day lost cannot be regained. Nagasena quotes:

> "Tis one night only, hunter, that we've spent
> Away from home, and that against our will,
> And thinking all night through of one another,
> Yet that one night is it that we bemoan,
> And grieve; for nevermore can it return."[10]

In the Vedic Aryan tradition we are told that the snake coils his body seven times in a spiral, a rhythmic circling indicative of the lunar tides of time—the tides of the ocean that come and go. The ocean of Divine Wisdom in the life of the individual has its own tides. Sometimes the waves may roll back, and the bare sand, stones, and shells become visible; they have been tossed by the power of the waves onto the shore. Yet that barrenness implies the coming of a new wave with even greater power, greater heights, to be followed by a roll of waves, one after the other. Year after year wintertime comes, harvest having taken place, and the land is barren. But invisible activities, similar to the waves, never cease. An aspirant will go through these phases also.

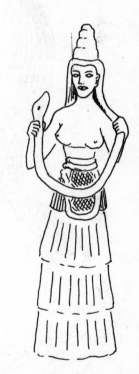

The cobra has to continually shed its skin in order to grow. How many times does an aspirant have to shed the old skin to let the new being emerge? Each time it is a mini-resurrection that will lead to a greater re-birth.

The snake is usually a symbol of fertility, contrary to the achievement of Higher Consciousness. But if the aspirant can follow the wise serpent, symbol of inner strength, it will present, silently and suddenly, awareness of the innate wisdom that has always been within, endowing the individual with the magnetic force of spiritual power.

Cretan serpent goddess of fertility

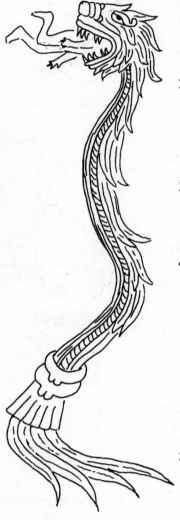

1. "In Greek mythology . . . the serpent represented the principle of life bound to the cycle of renewal, sloughing death." Campbell, *Occidental Mythology*, 259.

   The ouroboros, the mythological figure of a snake biting its own tail, is a symbol of self-renewing power in many cultures.

2. Quetzalcoatl, the plumed serpent god of Aztec Mexico, was a fertility god. Neumann, *The Great Mother*, 204.

   The snake goddess of Old Europe, represented in many forms, was also linked to fertility. In Crete she was known as a household goddess. Hutchinson, *Prehistoric Crete*, 108.

3. "The supporting energy and substance of the universe, and consequently of the individual, is imaged in India in the figure of the serpent. And the yogi is the master of this power." Campbell, *Primitive Mythology*, 436.

4. The waters of the Yamuna River had been poisoned by the black serpent, Kaliya, and all beings exposed to the water fell dead. Lord Krishna jumped into the river and, being a god, did not have to battle the serpent but sported with him instead. The outraged Kaliya whirled around himself in his attempt to overpower Krishna, but Krishna gracefully mounted the serpent's head and began to dance. Seeing his head being crushed by Krishna's dancing feet, Kaliya's wives begged Krishna to absolve their husband from his evil deeds. Krishna, in his compassion, granted their request and banished Kaliya to an island in the sea. *Bhagavata Purana*, X.16.

5. The serpent has been associated with the rainbow by the Greeks, the Chinese, the French, and the Africans among others. "The Celestial Serpent . . . symbolizes the rainbow and can form a bridge from this world to the next." Cooper, *Illustrated Encyclopaedia of Traditional Symbols*, 148-150.

6.   The crown of the Egyptians shows the head of a serpent and symbolizes, in a way that could hardly be better, the wisdom that comes from clear thinking, discrimination, courage, and the insight of the intuitive forces.

7.   Only a few people besides the snake charmer are interested enough in snakes to want to find out all about their behavior and their poison. Scientists have this kind of interest and it may be for this reason that the intertwining snakes of the caduceus became a symbol of medicine and healing in early times. Heinrich Zimmer traces the caduceus back to Mesopotamia where it was a symbol of the god of healing. Then it appeared in Greece as the healing god, Asklepios. Zimmer, *Myths and Symbols,* 74.

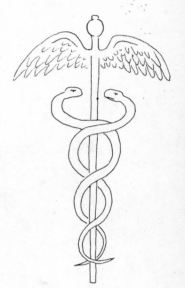

"The Greeks usually saw dreams as issuing from the underworld (a concept not unlike that of the unconscious mind) and so the snake, as inhabitant and symbol of that region, naturally became the symbol of the god who healed by dreams." *Encyclopedia of World Mythology,* 224.

The serpent power of the Kundalini system is symbolic for a different kind of healing—one in which the latent potential within each individual is actualized.

8.   Tawney, *Ocean of Story,* vol. 2, 312.

9.   The serpent power has a place in Western mythology as well. Joseph Campbell relates a story from Sumerian mythology in which King Gilgamesh was not satisfied with leading a life centered on the pleasures of the senses. He wanted something more, so he embarked upon a journey to seek immortality. He was told that he must pluck the "plant of immortality at the bottom of the cosmic sea." He succeeded in doing this, but on his way home a serpent, attracted by the scent of the plant, took it from Gilgamesh and consumed it. Thus the Serpent Power of Immortal Life, once a property of man, was taken away. *Occidental Mythology,* 92.

10.   *The Questions of King Milinda,* VII, 5, 23.

Kurma means "tortoise," and the final stage of the pose resembles a tortoise withdrawn into its shell. In the first stage, the legs are over the arms which are outstretched on either side of the body, chest and shoulders on the floor. In the next stage, the hands are brought behind the body palms up. In the final stage, Supta Kurmasana, the feet are crossed, the arms behind the back with the hands clasped, the forehead on the floor.

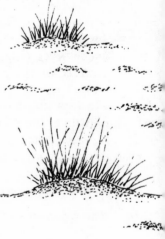

kurmasana
TORTOISE

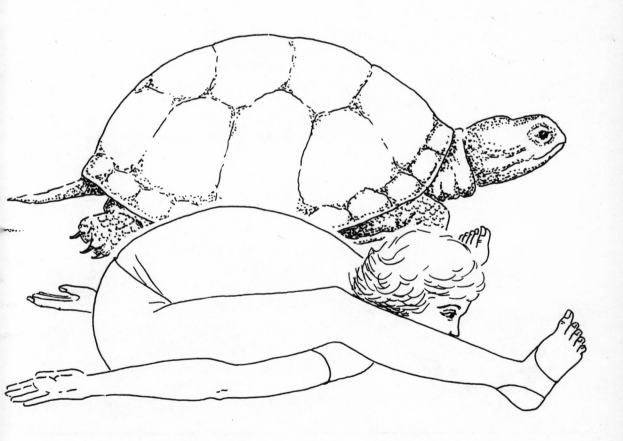

"You must develop character as the Kurma, the tortoise. When once it is in its shell, nothing at all can disturb it. In Kurmasana you are unable to see anyone or anything, obliging you to turn the attention inwards."
B.K.S. Iyengar

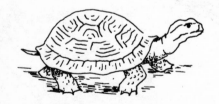

kurmasana

TORTOISE

THE CURVE OF THE SHELL of the tortoise is like the arc of the heavens; and the patterns on the shell have been associated with the night sky and its constellations of stars and planets. It reminds us of the search of the ancients to find meaning in the patterns of the stars with which to guide their lives. Human curiosity has to discover the secret behind markings of any kind. There is a fascination in deciphering the unknown, and joy in the victory of discovery.

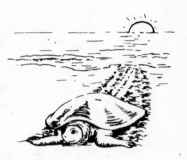

The tortoise and the sun, both rich in symbolism, have several things in common. The marks on the shell of the tortoise look like swirls of light, reminding one of the sun. The tortoise is slow-moving; the sun moves slowly across the horizon. There is a belief that the tortoise never gets lost; the sun also never gets lost. People in early days believed that, like the tortoise seeking a hiding place to rest, the sun also found its place of rest. The light of the day and its activity, and the darkness of the night providing rest, are perfectly balanced.

For many people Kurmasana is a difficult posture; preparatory practices are necessary before going into it. This emphasizes the need for the slow development of all asanas if they are to be experienced in depth. It is another reminder that, in the practice of asanas, competition has no place. The slowness, as symbolized by the tortoise, is objectionable only to the gross perception of the senses. Have I the patience to develop the flexibility to do this posture? Can I bend far enough? Will I ever find that inner place of rest?

KURMASANA: Tortoise Posture

Curve, arc of the heavens, patterns, search for meaning, curiosity, fascination, discovery, swirls of light, slow-moving, never gets lost, hiding place, balance, slow development, objectionable, difficulties, can't bend, tightness in my hips, where can I hide? where can I rest?

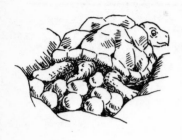

The tortoise lays several hundred eggs, which it does not look after; they are left to hatch by themselves. The eggs can be associated with ideas—some hatch and some simply die. Of the countless thoughts that pass through the mind, many are completely unnoticed; others are good ideas that seem, like the tortoise eggs, to hatch by themselves. Which of the many ideas are worth attending to? What is their nourishment?

There should not be too much emphasis placed on the method of performing the asana. The emphasis should rather be on the interplay between the body, the asana, and one's mental and emotional make-up: dependency, interdependency, and interaction. The asana then becomes a preparation for continuing self-investigation. One must learn all that is possible of the relationship between body and mind so they will work together rather than be in conflict. All movement of the body must be carefully considered and controlled, with full concentration on every muscle and on the breath. The asanas are designed in part to help the student become totally concentrated. These careful movements of the body have to spread into careful movements in all relationships.

E. A. Wallace Budge suggests that the powerful symbolic meaning of the tortoise may have come from Nubia where the Tortoise-god, Apesh, representing the powers of darkness and night, was revered out of fear.[1] Thought can be given to this ancient symbolism when doing the asana. Tight muscles, stiffness of the limbs, point to tensions that may reflect many fears. Fears can be based on a vividly stimulated imagination—which means there is no real basis for them. Fear creates unnecessary tension that manifests in the body in many ways. By directing the imagination, fearful ideas can be starved and thereby made to drop away. It is helpful to first make a list of all those that can be recognized, and then to weed them out. Memory reexamined reveals hidden fears; their power can be considerably diminished by prayer, Mantra, or meditation, which will help to shift focus.

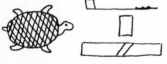

Tortoise-god Apesh

This asana makes one feel very vulnerable. With the arms and legs intertwined one cannot get up and run away from real or apparent danger, just as the tortoise does not run away but withdraws into its shell in a threatening situation. The basic response to fear is the desire for protection.

Ideas about protection are ambiguous, even though it is well-known that financial security, social position, and career success do not provide it. The need for protection is more powerful when emotions are threatened. To feel emotionally secure demands maturity, into which one can grow only slowly. The liberation of oneself from anxiety demands sharp observation and awareness.

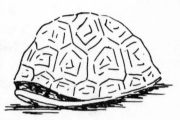

This does not exclude the necessity for occasionally retreating quickly into one's shell. Discrimination will teach when not to expose oneself unnecessarily to danger. Retreating into the shell can also help the quick- and hot-tempered person to become calm and composed.

The tortoise has a body which is, at the same time, soft and strong; the various situations which life presents demand that, with proper discrimination, we will sometimes be as strong as steel and at other times as soft as butter. The correct response will result in equanimity.

The aspirant must be careful not to intensify the shell for the purpose of keeping people from coming too close and intruding or touching. What is your shell made of: touchiness, defensiveness, irony, or sarcasm? To the degree in which these tendencies are present, they will reflect in the body. Physical and mental-emotional flexibility are interdependent.

KURMASANA: Tortoise Posture

Eggs, ideas, control, concentration, careful movements, tight muscles, stiffness, tension, fears, imagination, vulnerable, intertwined, shell, why do I withdraw?—from fear? for protection? retreating, intruding, touchiness, sensitivity, defensiveness

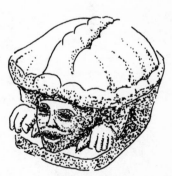

Aztec tortoise symbolizing bragging cowardice

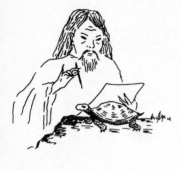

Symbolism changes from culture to culture, reflecting the needs of the people. Sometimes the tortoise has been endowed with the gift of prophecy, dispensing knowledge of the future as its most precious offering.[2] Prophecy has everywhere been greatly respected because of the common human characteristics of insecurity and fear. However, because men have decided women's way of life to a great extent, it is no surprise to find that they pointed to the tortoise as an example for women of chastity and refraining from idle talk. Pudicitia, a figure from Roman mythology, demonstrated these characteristics by putting her foot on the tortoise, because it never leaves its home (its shell) and does not talk.

In Egypt, the tortoise stood for fecundity, caution, and foresight. Being a water animal, it predicted through its behavior the rise of the Nile, fertilization of its shores, and production of food, thus granting the continuation of life. The intense desire for survival and longevity has been with the human race from the beginning, reflecting the awareness, however dim, that the purpose of each life is to come one step closer to remembering the divinity within.

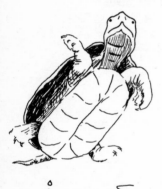

However, as every coin has two sides, there is also a speculation that the tortoise was an enemy of the god Ra. This is based on an inscription on a sarcophagus, "Ra liveth, the Tortoise dieth." The tortoise is also associated with the water god E-A, according to the interpretation of the constellation in the sky by the early Sumerians.

The *Bhagavad Gita* (II: 58) says, "When like the tortoise which withdraws on all sides its limbs, he (the aspirant) withdraws his senses from the sense-objects, then wisdom becomes steady." The tortoise symbolizes looking inward, and controlling very carefully what is put out.

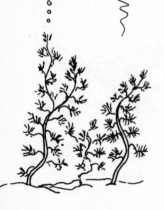

The perception of the world is only possible through the senses. Experience shows us the great difficulty there is in controlling sensory reactions and remaining neutral. Mind the interpreter is only too quick to color the message of the emotions, thereby reinforcing them. Temporarily retreating from all sense perceptions can restore or preserve the energy that is otherwise expended in argument, opposition, and the various expressions of opinion, all with little gain. Sensitive perception of the needs of others will help to overcome touchiness, which is a negative self-directed sensitivity. Argument can then become discussion, and confrontation can be directed toward self rather than against others.

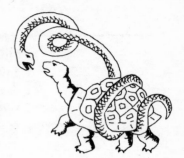

To stabilize emotions it is necessary to identify the personality aspect through which confrontation takes place. It is not possible to retreat from emotional influences entirely, but their compulsive effects can be minimized so that one becomes less vulnerable. Continuous reflection will bring about awareness of the wrong type of company and of undesirable influences which stimulate latent inclinations.

The tortoise lives near water and has to accept many strange creatures in its world of existence. When danger appears, the tortoise dives deep into the waters for safety. If the temptation of negative inclinations arises, the aspirant has to do the same thing—dive into the deep waters of meditation and withdraw all the senses to protect him or herself from being overtaken. Regular practice of meditation will give a sense of freedom from outside influences as well as from those negative characteristics that arise within.

Having withdrawn all its limbs, the tortoise will once again have to come out of its shell, return to living and finding food, and check to see if the bad company has disappeared. Discrimination is needed to decide when it is the right time to "stick one's neck out," to "stand up" (Tadasana) for oneself or others; or to know when it is the compulsive pressure of emotions that makes one charge ahead into affairs that are not one's responsibility. The ego will always be tempted to exert itself.

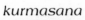

kurmasana

TORTOISE

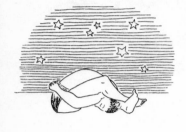

Four limbs and the head are exposed in this posture. There are supposedly five different pranic energies, even though they are all from the same source. There is a flow of mental energy as the thought of prana occurs. The purified mind could allow the flow of the prana to manifest in many parts of the body and many parts of your life.

What is in the mind of a tortoise? How little do we know! Human beings make greater and greater efforts to understand themselves and the world around, to find their place in the universe. If the shell of the tortoise is symbolic for the sky, where am I right now? What constellation is above me? Stars I cannot see, and yet I know they are there, becoming visible only at night. Is darkness necessary to make light and understanding desirable . . . even to bring longing?

REFLECTIONS: Tortoise

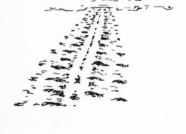

Human beings come into this world with the Divine Spark and a certain amount of conscience and awareness—limited, but sufficient to survive the adversity of an environment that is basically hostile to spiritual life. The shell of the tortoise, despite its advantage of protection, is not an easy thing to live with. Similarly, human beings find it difficult to live with awareness of the Divine Spark within; and this is obvious when we digress from proper conduct. Many people aspire to spiritual life but, in their pursuit of the divine goal, only a few are like the male sea turtle who goes into the surf after its birth, never to return to the land again.

Vivekananda, the first Indian yogi to come to America (at the end of the previous century), used the tortoise in his teachings and writings as a symbol to emphasize the necessity of overcoming obstacles, however great or painful. He pointed out that the tortoise, when it has withdrawn all its limbs, will not come out even if you put it into the fire and burn it.[3] For an aspirant to have that kind of strength and endurance to control all adverse influences that intrude from the outside world, and keep the inner forces intact, requires heroic effort. Only one who has an awareness of the powers of the Indriyas (senses) will not underestimate their ability to undermine the will and the best intentions.

The aspirant needs to beware of those who, with the clever use of the intellect in questioning the gain of spiritual life, can turn him or her upside down. It is useful to remember that when a tortoise is turned upside down it has not the power to turn back, so it dies. The seeker who gives a listening ear to the persuaders will thereby allow the Divine Spark within to die also. The temptations may be sweet at first but will leave a bitter taste, and memory will wrench the heart. The emptiness of a questionable future will not go away.

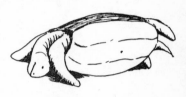

There are many delightful and charming Indian stories of the great flood that appears in so many different cultures. In India it has its culmination in the preserving aspect of the Hindu Trinity, Vishnu, who made it his responsibility to save the world. He became Kurma, the Great Tortoise, to carry the earth (Mount Mandara) on his back and prevent it from being swallowed by the churning waters. It seems that the earth has many times been in danger of being destroyed by turbulent waters. Vishnu is the compassionate aspect of the great creative power. He takes into consideration the frailty of the human race, which forgets its divine nature, that innate spark, and needs to be born again and again for another chance to undo whatever was wrong and to set it right.

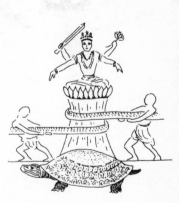

Vishnu and Mount Mandara on the back of Kurma

By using our personal power wisely, psychological obstacles disappear and our basic goodness, our ideals of ethics and loyalty, come into full play, leading to a contemplative way of life that will one day be crowned with Realization.

King Milinda pondered these serious questions, to which Nagasena had answers that were charming and yet deeply touching.[4] The king asked the sage to tell him the five qualities

TORTOISE

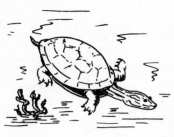

of the tortoise that every aspirant needs to attain. Nagasena answered that the first quality of the tortoise that a sincere aspirant must also have is that his heart must include the whole wide world with all its living creatures. And the heart must be filled with understanding and love, beyond measure of criticism or any feelings of hatred and malice—because the Life Force in all creatures is ONE.

The sage told also of another characteristic which the tortoise and seeker have in common. At the sight of approaching danger and temptation, the seeker lets himself sink into the depths of meditation, as the tortoise sinks into the depths of the water. Like the tortoise, the aspirant needs also to be in the sun, or the Light of knowledge and wisdom. While the tortoise would dig a hole in the ground to rest, the aspirant will retire to a quiet place for reflection and meditation.

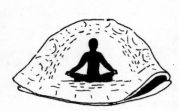

The ancient teachers were all aware that worldly gain, honor, and praise, had to be avoided. Inner quietness, reflection, and meditation can be found in solitude during a time set aside to be holy. A cave or little cottage in the mountains is helpful to break habits acquired in the city. Another option is to retreat into a room set aside for meditation. If all else fails, there is the cave of one's own heart and the invisible world where knowledge radiates from other sources.

Before the sage left, the king received a summary: "This, O king, is the fifth of the qualities of the tortoise that the aspirant ought to have. For it was said, O king, by the Blessed One, the god over all gods, in the most excellent Samyutta Nikaya, in the Sutta of the parable of the tortoise: 'As the tortoise withdraws his limbs in his shell, let the Bhikshu [aspirant] bury the thoughts of his mind, himself independent, injuring none, set free himself, speaking evil of none.'" [5]

All the great ones retreated from time to time into the shell of their innermost being, to seek that Divine Spark within, the spiritual gift from the Creative Power. When the aspirant looks with awe into the cave of the heart, the ego-mind (body-mind) has no choice but to retreat from the Light.[6]

Life is not a straight line; it is motion, and as such, it is a wave. When we look at the sky we see the curvature of the horizon, like the curve of the tortoise's shell, and we stand in awe of the flickering lights of the many stars and planets. Self-importance, the greatest obstacle that stands in the way of going beyond limitations, becomes like a grain of sand in the search for the answer to the recurring questions, Where is my place in the universe? What is my relationship to the cosmos? Who am I?

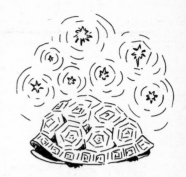

When you are able to take the tortoise position with ease, you may also have the relieving thought that, with all previous psychological problems off your chest, trust in yourself has significantly increased. And when you curve your back you might be reminded of the great tortoise, Kurma, who carried the earth, Mount Mandara, on his back.

The shell of the tortoise is its house and a permanent attachment. It has freedom and limitations at the same time. How wonderful it would be if one's temple of the Most High were such an attachment, making it impossible to step outside![7] This invokes a kind of independence for the aspirant that only a very few are able to achieve.

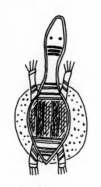

1. "It is not difficult to see why the tortoise should have gained the reputation he bears in African and other folklore. His ability to exist for a long time without food, the difficulty of killing him, the ease with which he conceals himself, together with his slow movements and uncanny appearance all combine to suggest infinite watchfulness, patience, endurance, and wisdom, a grim sense of humour, and magical or preternatural powers of some sort." Maculloch, *The Mythology of All Races,* vol. 7, 309.

2. "There were religious ceremonies in ancient China in which the tortoise was placed in front of all the other offerings because of its knowledge of the future." *Li Ki,* VII.II, 17.

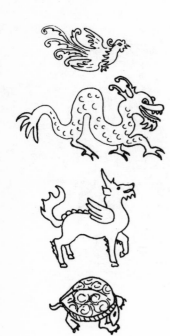

The tortoise was also believed to be highly intelligent: "What were the four intelligent creatures? They were the *Khi*-lin, the phoenix, the tortoise, and the dragon. When the dragon becomes a domestic animal, (all other) fishes and the sturgeon do not lie hidden from men (in the mud). When the phoenix becomes so, the birds do not fly from them in terror. When the *Khi*-lin does so, the beasts do not scamper away. When the tortoise does so, the feelings of men take no erroneous course.' (Translator's note: "The lesson drawn from the text by many is that men's goodness is the pledge of, and the way to, all prosperity.") Ibid.,VII.IV, 10.

3. "As the tortoise tucks its feet and head inside the shell, and you may kill it and break it in pieces, and yet it will not come out, even so the character of that man who has control over his motives and organs is unchangeably established. He controls his own inner forces, and nothing can draw them out against his will. By this continuous reflex of good thoughts, good impressions moving over the surface of the mind, the tendency for doing good becomes strong, and as the result we feel able to control the Indriyas (the sense organs, the nerve-centres)." Swami Vivekananda, *Karma Yoga,* 40.

4. *The Questions of King Milinda,* VII, 1, 12. (See also VII, 6, 3.)

5. Ibid., VII, 1, 16.

6. The phrases "to be reborn" (Jesus), "born of," or "giving birth to" from the various schools of thought, very aptly describe what takes place. Birth is given to the being of Light within oneself, an event of indescribable beauty, although the experiences gained can often be a bit disconcerting. The gestation period, during which the limitations imposed by psychological problems are transcended, is, of course, not painless. But then suddenly one sees the wild flowers that before were too small, too modest, to be noticed on a walk through the meadow. Suddenly the bird's song in the early morning is music to one's ears, whereas before it may have been an annoyance, disturbing anticipated hours of sleep. One is born into a new life. The questions then arise, Am I a god or goddess in human likeness, or a human being in divine likeness? If the Kingdom of God is within, am I called upon to be its ruler?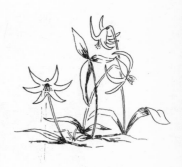

That glimpse, that fleeting moment, that breath of freedom, can become a shining jewel in the depths of your memory. From there it can generate Light and power to propel a heartfelt desire for freedom and Liberation.

7. "That lower shell of it is this terrestrial world; it is, as it were, fixed; for the fixed, as it were, is this earth-world. And that upper shell of it is yonder sky; it has its ends, as it were, bent down; for yonder sky has its ends, as it were, bent down. And what is between the shells is the air. That tortoise thus is these worlds; it is these worlds he thus lays down to form part of the altar." *Satapatha Brahmana,* part VII:5, 1.

kurmasana

TORTOISE

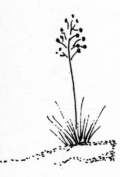

Vrishchika means "scorpion," the creature this pose resembles. With the forearms resting on the floor, the legs are raised up, and the head and chest lifted. The legs are bent at the knees, and the feet lowered slowly behind the back until they rest on the crown of the head.

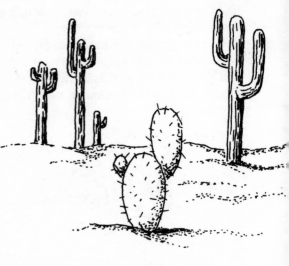

vrishchikasana

SCORPION

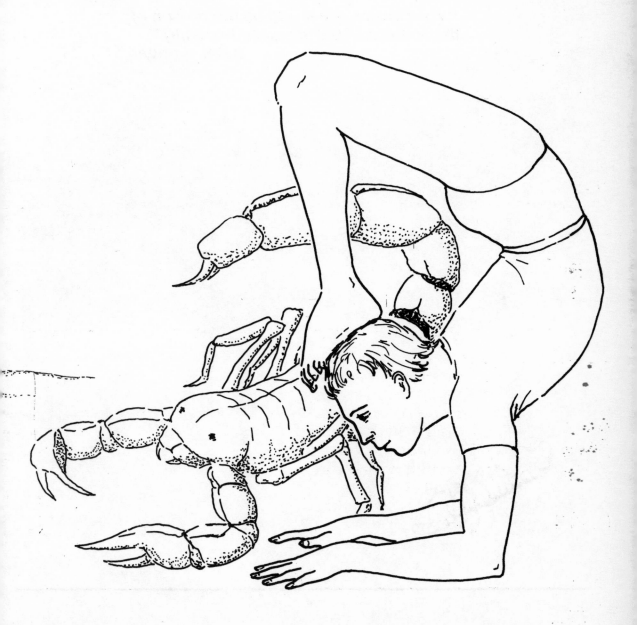

"Your brains are stung by the poison of the scorpion—the scorpion is vanity."
B.K.S. Iyengar

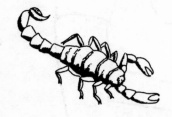

vrishchikasana

SCORPION

THE SCORPION IS a dangerous creature, easily excited, responding with lightning swiftness to the slightest movement, attacking without proper discrimination.[1] When the scorpion stings, it is the powerful poison that it emits that creates pain. The poison has a tremendously potent effect on the nervous system, and people scream for days in great pain.

The lovely Egyptian goddess, Selket, stands with arms outstretched in a protective gesture in the tomb of the Pharaoh.[2] She wears on her head, like a crown, a scorpion whose sting she is able to counteract with her magic. What does it mean to put a crown on your head? Is it glorification of the ego? In the Kundalini system, the crown with many colors and many jewels is glorifying Consciousness, also symbolized by the diamond reflecting different lights from different facets.

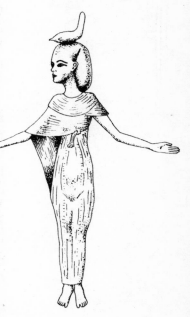

In Vrishchikasana, the pelvic area is lifted off the ground so that there is an even greater need for balance, skill, and strength than in doing the headstand. In this position also, one can receive the nectar and ambrosia (intuitive insights) and feel a longing for the glorifying of Consciousness. When we allow the Divine Forces to sting our self-glorification, we receive a reward beyond all expectations.

What does it mean to do this asana? Why would it be called "scorpion"? Am I stinging people to hurt them? Or would I like to have the sensitivity to respond with a scorpion-like quickness to even an unspoken need? Can I show compassion without waiting for someone to beg on their knees? Jesus said when someone asks you to walk a mile, go a second mile. Do I respond to the need of people with this kind of generosity, or do I speculate whether the individual is worth my time?

VRISHCHIKASANA: Scorpion Posture

Dangerous, without proper discrimination, stings, pain, potent, protective, magic, crown, balance, skill, strength, nectar and ambrosia, glorifying of Consciousness, self-glorification, reward, sting to hurt, compassion, generosity, worth my time, sexual activity

First there may be the realization of the many stings by which other people have been hurt. Then comes the understanding that personal suffering is the result of the previously unnoticed attachments and self-importance receiving a sting from the Divine.

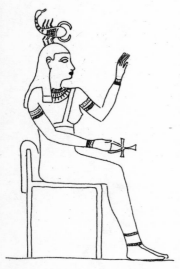

The compassion of the goddess Selket is offered for all women, from the poorest peasant to the reigning queen. She gives health and assistance in childbirth, and fills other needs when her worshippers turn to her. She is willing to rescue women from ignorance and help them to become aware of their divine potential. This is the same compassion that we see in the Virgin Mary, in Tara of the Tibetan Buddhists, and in Kwan Yin in China or Japan. They know of the incredible temptation of the forces of nature and procreation, and what it takes for consciousness to overcome instincts.

The relationship of the sting of the scorpion to sexual activity can be easily understood as the sting of the male to the female. For the man the choice is not any different than for the woman: to procreate either by penetrating the womb of a female to deposit the seed (for which in the Old Testament he is called "the seeder"), or by penetrating the womb of Divine Wisdom and surrendering all his instinctual forces to Divine Mother. Then he will receive from her the gift of inner sight, the ability to hear with the third ear, and the ability to discriminate between the experience of physical pleasure and that of spiritual ecstasy.

Divine Mother will never let her devotee down. May you find her in the tabernacle of your consciousness.

1. The scorpion's vicious nature gave it the reputation in ancient Egypt of being the protector of evil and darkness. Churchward, *Signs and Symbols of Primordial Man*, 103.

2. Selket is one of four goddesses whose elegant statues guard the tomb of Tutankhamun.

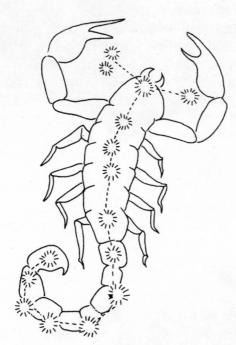

The constellation Scorpius

BIRDS

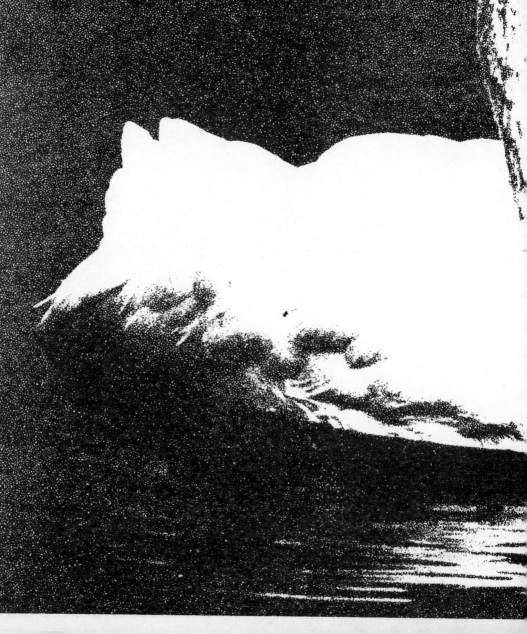

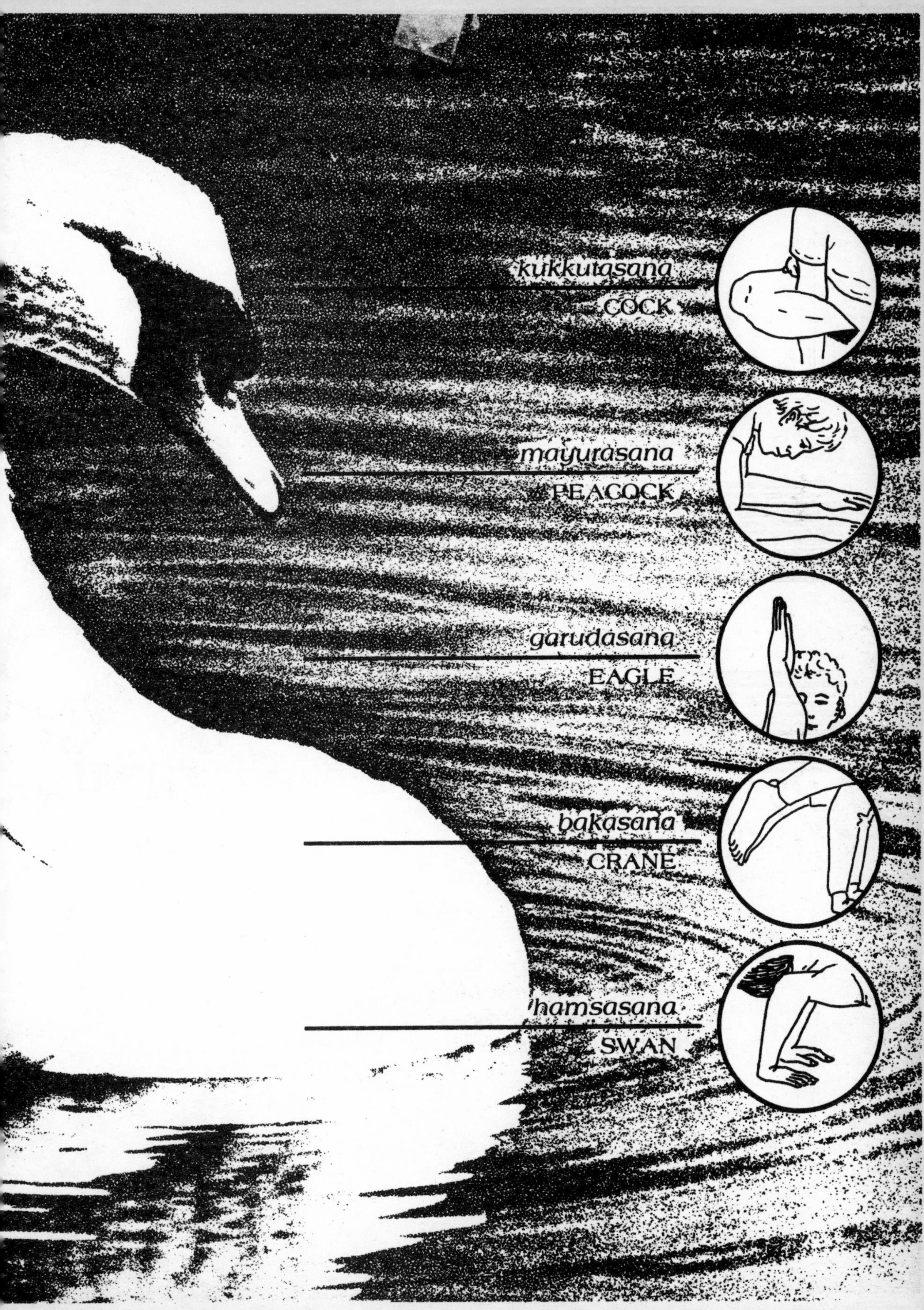

kukkutasana
COCK

mayurasana
PEACOCK

garudasana
EAGLE

bakasana
CRANE

hamsasana
SWAN

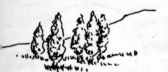

Kukkuta means "cock." With the legs crossed in Padmasana, the hands and arms are placed between the calf and thigh of each leg, and the body is raised off the floor in a position that resembles a cock. The pose is repeated with the legs crossed in the opposite way.

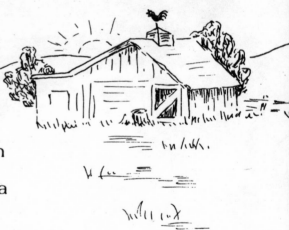

kukkutasana

COCK

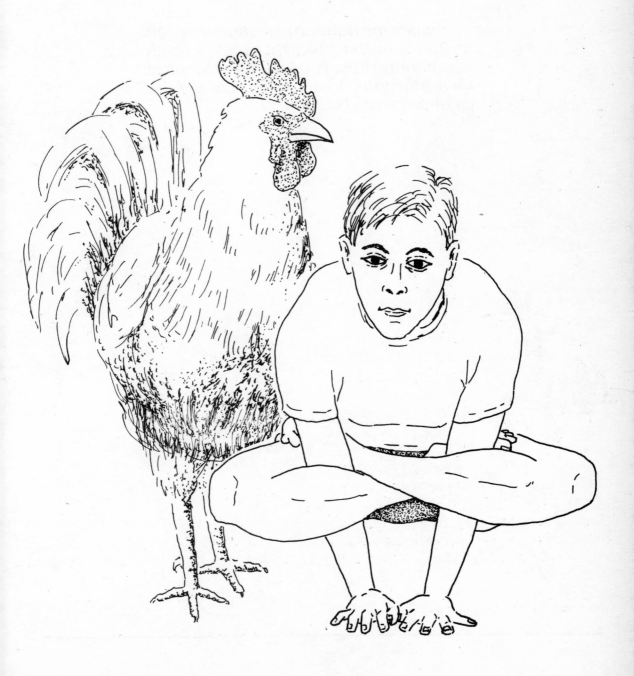

"Awaken the dormant intelligence even in the minutest fibre; this will help its neighboring fibres to revitalise, to realize their functions, to act, to experience the creation created by you."

B.K.S. Iyengar

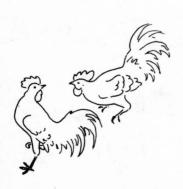

kukkutasana

COCK

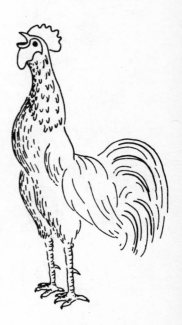

Bɪʀᴅs ᴄᴀɴ ʙᴇ sᴇᴇɴ as focal points for human emotions, habits, and attitudes. Symbolism, as we have already seen, has a nearly inexhaustible repertoire. The symbol, when taken out of its narrow context, is an important tool to convey or teach subtleties otherwise lost in logic; however, sheer literal-mindedness in the interpretation of symbols is sometimes practical and valuable when a more sophisticated interpretation could add to existing confusion.

An interesting Greek story explains why the cock crows at sunrise. Mars wanted to spend the night with Venus while her husband, Vulcan, was away. He commissioned Alektraon to watch at the door but he fell asleep, and Vulcan arrived home and surprised the couple. Mars punished Alektraon by turning him into a cock, the herald of the dawn. This quality of vigilance, which Alektraon lacked, is essential to the aspirant's spiritual life. It is also essential in the execution of the posture, Kukkutasana.

Kukkutasana does look very much like a cock, and it is not as difficult as it appears, although it calls for great strength in the wrists and hands, and flexibility in the legs. This challenging asana also requires a good sense of balance and breath control, total concentration, and vigilance. Have I the concentration to balance on my hands? It takes courage to maintain balance. Are my arms strong enough to hold me? Will my legs stay in place?

KUKKUTASANA: Cock Posture
Emotions, habits, attitudes, strength, flexibility, balance, breath control, concentration, vigilance; feeling restricted, locked in, unsteady, what if I fall on my face? can't go anywhere, what can I see from here? where shall I focus my attention?

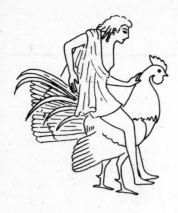

In Greek mythology the cock was sacred to Apollo, god of the sun, and was associated with Asclepius, Apollo's son and the god of healing. In fact, cocks were sacrificed to Asclepius when a person recovered from an illness. The crowing cock puts demons to flight in the Persian *Zend-Avesta*. Yet for the Celts he is a symbol of lust and adultery, incest, egotism, and defiance. In Rome he was considered an oracle, predicting the outcome of war by the way he would crow in the morning. According to Pliny, even the lions are afraid of him. There is great diversity in the symbolism of the cock. It seems to express the pairs of opposites which the aspirant must deal with in life.

Two fighting cocks on the tombs of Christians represented courage under persecution. The cock is famous in Christian iconography because, after it had crowed thrice, Peter realized that he had denied his Master. In folklore he is the animal who is supposed to have announced the birth of Christ. Was the cock a prophet, a devil's messenger, or was he, as the Scandinavians claim, charged with wakening and speeding forth the heroes?

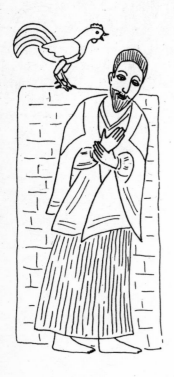

The cock was associated with the sun in almost all religions. The Chinese believed that it was the cock's well-accepted duty to awaken the glorious sun and thereby dispel darkness, which also signaled that the evil spirits of the night who fear the bright light would be kept away. The cock within the aspirant awakens the spiritual sun which drives away the forces of darkness.

In China, the cock is the primary symbol for the element of *yang,* the masculine principle, representing the warmth and life of the universe. The Chinese also endow the cock with five virtues. The crown on his head symbolizes a literary spirit, while the spurs on his feet show his warlike disposition and courage. But he is also benevolent, clucking for his hens when he finds delicious food to share; and his faithfulness is shown by the reliability with which he crows to herald the day.

When in this posture, as you ponder the implications of the cock in various mythologies, you might also consider the characteristic of cockiness. Am I so cocksure that I overlook the need for strength and balance? Do pride and arrogance override flexibility, poise, and benevolence? When does courage become aggression? Can I remain immobile and just survey my territory?

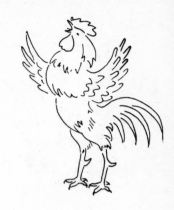

KUKKUTASANA: Cock Posture

Healing, lust, egotism, defiance, sacrifice, courage, denial, prophet, devil's messenger, awakening the sun, evil spirits, yang, masculine, literary spirit, warlike disposition, benevolence, faithfulness, cockiness

There is no doubt that the cock is in control of the flock. He dominates his hens, as well as fertilizing their eggs. He will protect his own hens when he thinks something unpleasant is going to happen, and will make an awful racket to drive away an intruder. This protective aspect of the cock could include jealousy.

Each cock has his own personality aspects. One will eat first and pay no attention to whether there is enough food for the hens. Another will let the hens feed first, and eat later himself. He may also have a special communication with his favorite hen, and share his food with her.

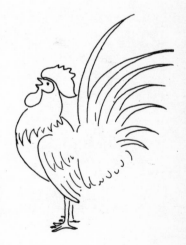

Although the cock is noted for strutting, in this posture very little movement is possible. Does pride lock me into position? Maybe I need to stop for awhile and look at my personality aspects so I can use my strength in a better way, showing care and concern for others.

King Milinda and Nagasena had a conversation about the five qualities in the cock that an aspirant should emulate. First, the cock goes early to roost at the end of the day, and the aspirant, when he has completed his duties, should retire early.

Second, the aspirant, like the cock, rises early in the morning to sweep out the open space, readying the drinking water for the day's use; after he has taken his bath, he dresses himself before he goes to bow down in reverence before the Master; then he pays a visit to the senior aspirants and returns to enter again his solitude.

Third, the cock is unremitting in scratching the earth to find what he can to eat; and so the sincere aspirant should practice continual self-examination and circumspection, in taking any nourishment that can be found to eat, and remembering "I eat this, seeking not after pleasure nor excitement, nor beauty of body, nor after elegance of form, but merely for the preservation of my body, to keep myself alive, as a means of appeasing the pain of hunger, and of assisting me in the practice of the higher life. Thus shall I put an end to all former sorrow, and give no cause for future sorrow to arise."[1]

Fourth, as the cock has eyes to see and yet is blind at night, the earnest aspirant also should be blind to the temptation of the senses. Fifth, the cock, even though persecuted, will not leave his home, and the sincere aspirant, regardless of his daily duties in making robes, building shelter, and everything that is demanded of him, will never give up his presence of mind—the home in which he dwells.

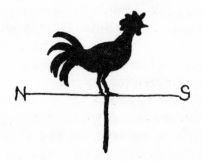

kukkutasana

COCK

1.   *Questions of King Milinda,* VII, 1, 3.

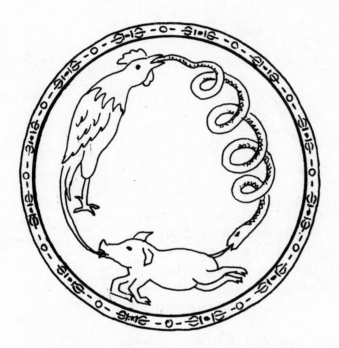

At the center of the Tibetan Wheel of Life are three animals: a cock, a snake, and a pig or boar. These animals represent the "three poisons" or primary motivating forces of the ego: greed, hate, and delusion. They are shown biting each others' tails, a symbolic representation of the way in which these negative aspects feed on themselves.

kukkutasana

COCK

Mayura means "peacock." In this pose, the hands are placed on the floor facing backward with the little fingers touching. The body is lifted up parallel to the floor, the upper arms supporting the chest.

Pincha Mayurasana is the peacock feather pose. The forearms and hands are placed firmly on the floor, the head raised. The legs are lifted up so that torso and legs are perpendicular to the floor. The pose resembles a peacock feather or a peacock with its tail raised.

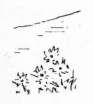

mayurasana
PEACOCK

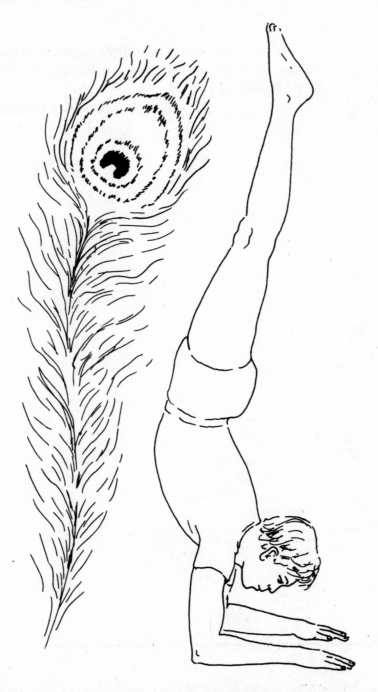

"As beginners our intellect is only in the brain. You must have a million eyes, all over the body."

B.K.S. Iyengar

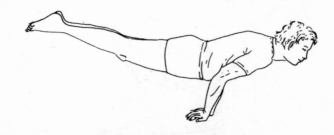

mayurasana

PEACOCK

THE PEACOCK IS ASSOCIATED with many deities of the
[Ea]st, but it has also been used as a symbol in the Western
[w]orld. It has gone by many names, such as the Persian Bird, or
[th]e bird of Kwan Yin and Amitabha. It is also called Juno's
[bi]rd by the Romans, and is Hera's bird in Greek mythology. To
[sit] on a peacock throne, like the Persian royal throne, must
[in]deed be a majestic feeling.

The peacock with its beautiful crown is the emblem of
[Sa]raswati, the Indian goddess of wisdom, music, and poetry.
[E]ven Lakshmi, the goddess of wealth and plenty, avails herself
[of] a peacock to ride. Brahma uses the majestic peacock as a
[ve]hicle, and Lord Krishna carries on his head the feather of this
[ex]otic-looking bird. This bird of kings and gods is a suitable
[sy]mbol for the aspirant's striving for the highest.

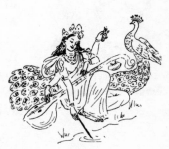

Saraswati

The bird itself is known to be an effective killer of snakes.
[It] can also be quarrelsome, moody, and unpredictable, even
[to]ward those who feed it. But it is certainly beauty that gives
[th]e peacock its fame. All the peacock's movements, although
[th]ey may look frivolous, are part of its mating ritual. The
[be]autiful tail fan, which he unfolds during courting, appears to
[th]e female only as a flag that stimulates her responses.

There is no question that the peacock is one of the most
[ad]mired birds because of the beauty of its iridescent blue tail
[fe]athers. It is probably human speculation that the bird knows
[its] tail to be of exquisite beauty, and therefore gives way to
[pr]ide in appearance. However, the interpretation of the pea-
[co]ck as standing for worldliness, pride, and vanity, has fre-
[qu]ently been used in Christian stories.[1] It is said that when the
[bi]rd sees its feet, it screams, realizing how ugly they are in
[co]ntrast to its beautiful plumage. Does pride blind me to my
[ug]ly side? Or does it make me oversensitive to my imperfec-
[ti]ons? Can beauty be a symbol of my aspirations, of perfection

beyond the worldly kind? To reach that perfection I have to strengthen my arms—they are not stable enough to hold my weight.

MAYURASANA: Peacock Posture

Royal, majestic, wisdom, music, poetry, wealth, exotic, kings and gods, striving, killer, quarrelsome, moody, unpredictable, ritual, beauty, iridescence, exquisite, worldliness, pride, vanity, weak in arms and wrists, not very stable, where will I find perfection? can see no beauty in this position

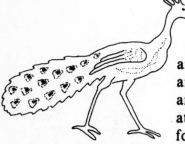

Mosaic detail from sixth century Christian art

The peacock was taken over from pagan into Christian art, where it symbolizes the resurrection, the beauty of the soul, and the many graces that are bestowed in the sacrament. There are examples in the Roman catacombs and also in the baptistry at Naples. The peacock was the only bird that did not eat of the forbidden fruit in the Garden of Eden. It was rewarded, according to an old Jewish legend, with eternal life, thereby becoming the mystical bird, the phoenix, signifying resurrection, rebirth, and a vision of eternity.

Darwin drew the conclusion that the attraction of one living being for another is a mighty influence on evolution, and that beauty outweighs even success in battle—a fact that has been well-proven in humans also. Beautiful people find more acceptance, and their pride and arrogance is taken more kindly, while those who are not pleasing to the eye, although they may possess a brilliant mind and positive characteristics such as kindness, take longer to be accepted.

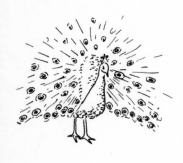

Mayurasana demands great strength in the wrists and arms, and a tuning into the balance of the body; so the hundred eyes of the peacock's tail point to vigilance rather than to beauty. There is little room for vanity when the weight of the whole body is carried on the small area of the hands. Facing downward, the eyes can only look at a small area on the ground. One is reminded of the watchfulness and compassion of the Buddhist Avalokitesvara, or Amitabha, who has the peacock feather as an attribute.

The peacock may be a quarrelsome bird, cackling and strutting, but the asana points to a wise choice between pride or arrogance, and the potential that is perhaps symbolized in the beauty of the peacock's tail fan.

MAYURASANA: Peacock Posture

Resurrection, many graces, reward, mystical, rebirth, vision of eternity, attraction, acceptance, tuning, watchfulness, compassion, quarrelsome, cackling, strutting, pride, arrogance, potential, choice, paradox, promise

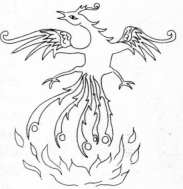

The peacock and the phoenix are closely related, both being symbols of resurrection and immortality.[2] But it is only the phoenix who will die by self-immolation. There have been yogis who, withdrawing the life force, immolated their bodies. In modern times there have been those who have burnt their bodies as a means of protest. There is the Indian widow who, believing in rebirth, follows her husband into death, and the Japanese *kamikasi* (soldier) who will set a bomb and blow himself up with it. All find the expression of their ideal in the beautiful peacock/phoenix.

When the phoenix has been burned, from the ashes there emerges a new phoenix, resurrected to begin life again, symbolizing that when ignorance is burned in the fire of wisdom, mental and spiritual rebirth takes place.

These two birds, the peacock and phoenix, are also associated with the *yin-yang.* In the white part of that symbol there is already the seed of destruction or decay; in the black there is the seed, a white dot, indicating rebirth, a new life, new construction. It is said that when either the hen or peacock of a couple dies, the other cannot live long—again reflecting the yin-yang interdependence.

The peacock has many other associations. The beautiful iridescent colors of its tail are connected with the worship of

PEACOCK

the sun[3] and, of course, with love, with the promises made in the unfolding of the feathers during the mating dance. The peacock is associated with the tree, and with the stars of the solar system, as longevity and immortality. The phoenix also is a celestial symbol of a cyclic period, whose brightest star is Ankaa, which is ninety-three light-years away. In the lands of the Nile this "sun bird" is supposed to have a period of 500 to 1,000 years before it arises from its own ashes to a new life once again.

The paradox of the symbolism of the peacock is evident in the posture. It is a difficult one for many people; one must overcome pride, bodily fear, fear of not completing the pose, of not being able to do the right thing, fear of showing weakness. And yet, the beauty in the spread of the tail holds out a promise. Even a single feather represents the third eye of all-knowledge and heavenly Light.[4] The spread of the tail of the peacock is an incomplete circle. This shows that we can never see everything at once; we can see only the top, which is comparable to the first state of realization. Because the peacock stays on the ground, rather than flying, it represents the earth with all its colorful temptations. But the phoenix rising out of its own ashes is a symbol of the resurrection of which everyone is capable.

mayurasana

PEACOCK

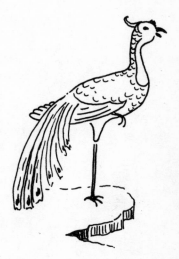

"It is commonly said of the peacock that it has an angel's feathers, a devil's voice, and a thief's walk." Gubernatis, *Zoological Mythology,* vol. 2, 324.

"The peacock, which annually loses and renews its various colours and splendours, and is fruitful in progeny, served, like the phoenix, as a symbol of immortality, and a personification of the fact that the sky is obscured and becomes serene again, that the sun dies and is born again, that the moon rises, is obscured, goes down, is concealed, and rises once more." Ibid., 327.

"The serene and starry sky and the shining sun are peacocks. The calm azure heavens, bespangled with a thousand stars, a thousand brilliant eyes and the sun rich with the colours of the rainbow, offer the appearance of a peacock in all the splendour of its eye besprinkled feathers." Ibid., 323.

Joseph Campbell refers to the eyes of the peacock feathers as being equivalent to the eye in the middle of the forehead, "which opens in man to the vision of eternity." See *The Masks of God: Creative Mythology,* 503.

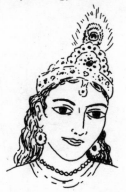

Krishna wearing the peacock feather in his crown

Garuda is the eagle, the king of birds and the vehicle of Vishnu. This pose requires great concentration and balance as the weight is entirely on one leg with the thigh of the other leg in front, the lower leg behind, and the toes around the inner side of the ankle of the standing leg. The upper arms are held forward and parallel to the floor, with the forearms twisted around each other so that the palms of the hands are together. The pose is repeated standing on the other leg, the arms reversed.

garudasana

EAGLE

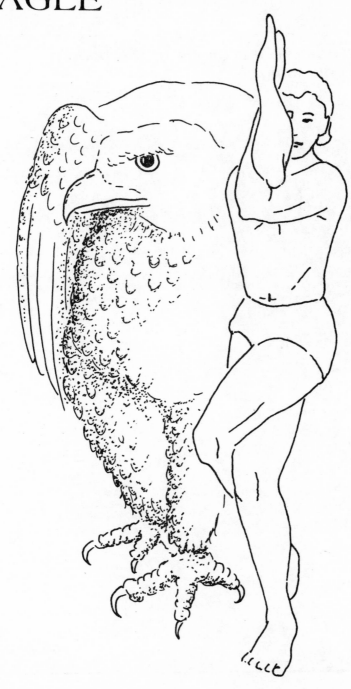

*"The ribs are the wings of the body.
Open your wings."*

B.K.S. Iyengar

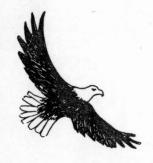

garudasana

EAGLE

THE EAGLE IS THE KING of the birds, a symbol of power and victory. A bird of prey, it hunts from sunrise to sunset, flying and soaring over its territory, spotting faraway prey with its extremely keen eyesight. It strikes with such unerring accuracy that it has no enemies and it lives in solitary splendor. It is no surprise then that the eagle is an emblem of victory in battle and also of the triumph of spirit over intellect.

Eagles are symbolic for sharp sight, for penetrating vision.[1] If you can see through yourself, how you lay your own traps, you can avoid them. Because the eagle has clear sight, it can recognize things from a distance in time to take action.[2] The eagle flies around, watching, and knows precisely what it is aiming at when it dives for its prey. Questions like these, while trying Garudasana, will help you gain an eagle's perspective: Can I see through my traps? Can I avoid getting caught in them? What am I aiming at?

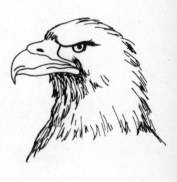

GARUDASANA: Eagle Posture
Power, victory, flying, soaring, hunting, keen eyesight, spirit over intellect, recognizing, watching, aiming, diving; twisting legs and arms, I feel like a pretzel; trapped, wound up—ready to spring into action? swaying, losing balance, need to focus, where is my focus?

Many cultures have associated the eagle with the most important of their gods. In Egypt, the solar symbolism was shared by the falcon and the eagle, and this heavenly principle is the divine vision that the aspirant seeks.[3] Ra, god of the Rising Sun, is often shown as falcon-headed, and Horus, the All-Seeing, appears either as a falcon or falcon-headed. The soul or essence (Ba) was represented by the Egyptians as a bird—probably a falcon—with a human head.

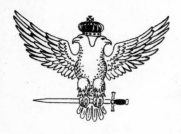

You can see the implications in Scandinavian mythology of Odin, the supreme god, changing into a falcon to travel to earth. The Greeks chose the eagle to be Zeus' bird, bearer of the thunderbolt and lightning; and for the Incas this bird is a solar symbol and, at the same time, a guardian spirit.

The aspirant might look at the aggressive qualities of the eagle, which was frequently used to symbolize supremacy and war. The first to carry the double-headed eagle on their standards were the Hittites. Other cultures adopted it,[4] and even in modern times, Austria has the double-headed eagle as its special emblem. The United States, the most powerful nation in the world today, uses the eagle as its symbol. The arms of Mexico show the eagle with the serpent, perhaps portraying life's opposites as supernatural power and victory in warfare.

According to an ancient Squamish legend the eagle was instrumental in bringing the salmon to Squamish waters. The American Indians also wear the enormous and impressive feather headdress of the Thunder Bird, representing the universal spirit. The East Indians have assigned the eagle to be the messenger of Indra, the god of the heavens. Sometimes the eagle is compared to the great mystical bird, Garuda (from which this posture derives its name). In *The Ocean of Story,* a collection of ancient Eastern myths, we are told that "the Garuda bird is the vehicle of Vishnu. It is described as half-man and half-bird, having the head, wings, beak and talons of an eagle, and human body and limbs."[5] Garuda attacks and destroys evil in the form of serpents. Once again this depicts the age-old conflict between power of mind or supreme intellect (the soaring eagle), and matter, temptation by the forces of the earth (the snake).

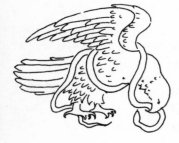

In all of us the conflict between the eagle (the spiritual) and the snake (temptation) is the ongoing struggle. Can I see my struggle clearly? What is my target? Can I soar like an eagle above the temptations of life?

When doing this asana, you can use the symbolism of the myths to expand your vision and understanding. You may be able to see clearly your own errors and what you can do differently. Such questions as these might come into your mind: What are my past errors? What are my victories? Human learning is usually through trial and error, but this asana offers an opportunity to gain a perspective that will diminish errors.

GARUDASANA: Eagle Posture

Heavenly principle, divine vision, all-seeing, guardian spirit, aggressive, supernatural power, victory in warfare, temptation, see through myself, trial and error, single-pointedness, visionary

Balance in this position is difficult—"I feel awkward, unsteady, tied in knots." And yet, when this posture is achieved, it is possible to concentrate with a single-pointedness that is like the clarity of the eagle's vision.

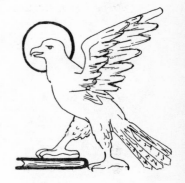

Today the person of outstanding intelligence, who has lofty thoughts and conceives of high-flying projects, is often compared to an eagle—someone above the average, the eagle of a group. The evangelist John, writer of the fourth gospel, is symbolized by the eagle because he was a visionary. The person who has clear sight and can see through things may turn this inward and learn by self-observation rather than by trial and error.

Aristotle tells a story of the eagle's fabulous eyesight which allowed it to look directly at the sun.[6] This story was later expanded to mean that Christ was the eagle who could look directly at his Father. In Jungian psychology, the story of Aphrodite and Psyche expresses the importance of having a panoramic vision like the eagle's, and of looking at the vast river of life for a greater perspective and expanded possibilities.

Nagasena uses the story of the generosity of a king called Vessantara to illustrate that, as long as we are on this earth, absolutes are not possible. Even the great eagle, Garuda,

symbol of divine vision, was overcome by Vessantara's goodnes[s].
King Milinda is told by Nagasena,

> [i]n the case of the splendid gift of Vessantara the glorious
> king, . . . [i]t is when overborne by the weight of right-
> eousness, overpowered by the burden of the goodness
> of acts which testify of absolute purity, that, unable to
> support it, the broad earth quakes and trembles and is
> moved. . . . He had abandoned, O king, all seeking after
> the craving after a future life, his strenuous effort was set
> only towards a higher life. . . . When he was thus giving
> away . . . the great winds began to blow confusedly . . . and
> at the movement of the waters the great fish and the scaly
> creatures were disturbed . . . and the Asuras, and Garudas,
> and Yakkhas, and Nagas shook with fear. [From: the
> dilemma as to the earthquake at Vessantara's gift.][7]

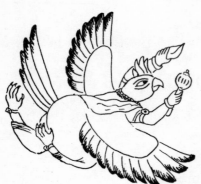

The Eagle, Garuda

Nagasena's words make it quite clear that no one can liv[e]
in absolute righteousness, absolute goodness, and absolut[e]
purity; because those absolutes would not be recognizab[le]
were it not for their opposites—the earthquakes within one['s]
own consciousness and the powerful waves of the waters [of]
emotions. There is the light of the day from the life-giving su[n]
and in the darkness of night there must be rest.

1. "In the iconography of the Four Elements in certain late medieval manuscripts, as the bird of Jove who lived in the heavens and as the symbol of St. John, . . . the eagle represented the element Air. In the presentation of the Five Senses, the eagle was the attribute of Sight." Rowland, *Birds With Human Souls,* 55.

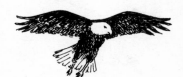

2. "An individual encountering the river of life from the narrow perspective of his own particular river bank may occasionally need to call on his eagle nature to lift his range of vision to take in more of the river, to see all the curves and turns and changes. Then he may put his own situation into better perspective and see other possibilities." Johnson, *She,* 58.

3. North American Indians also use the eagle in their reverence of the sun: "Dancers wear and use whistles made of the wing-bone of the eagle to which eagle plumes are attached. In recreating the cry of eagle to the powerful rhythm of song, dance, and

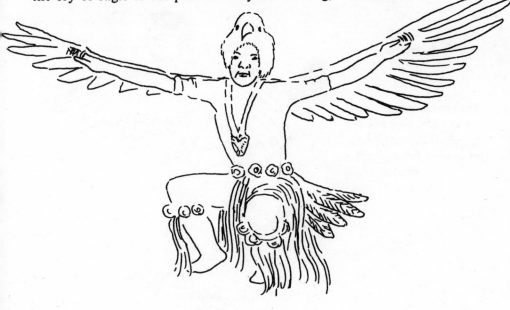

garudasana

EAGLE

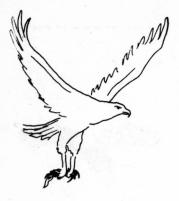

drum, the Eagle is present in voice and being, man's vital breath is united with the essence of sun and life. Through such ritual use of sacred form man becomes Eagle, and the eagle in his plumes is the Sun." Epes, "Sun dance: sacrifice, renewal, identity," 15.

4.   In Siberia "Yakut shamans and blacksmiths of the Turukhansk region pray especially to Ai Toyon, Creator of Light. He takes the form of a huge, radiant two-headed eagle, perched at the very tip of the world tree. From Ai Toyon's wide-spreading, snow-white pinions, physical light and the light of knowledge alike descend to earth. When shamans dream, Ai Toyon descends upon them." Eliot, *Myths,* 124.

5.   Tawney, *Ocean of Story,* vol. 1, 108.

6.   According to this story, the eagle forces its offspring to look at the sun and rejects those who are unable to do so. Rowland, *Birds With Human Souls,* 52.

7.   *Questions of King Milinda,* IV, 1, 37.

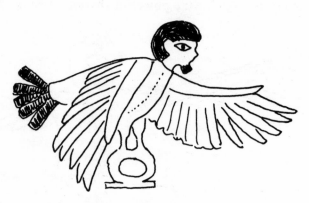

The soul or essence (Ba) was represented by the Egyptians as a bird, probably a falcon, with a human head.

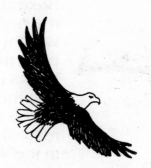

garudasana

EAGLE

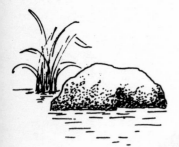

Baka means "crane." In this pose, the hands and arms support the weight of the body. The legs are bent, the shins resting on the backs of the upper arms, the feet together below the buttocks and off the ground. This pose resembles a crane wading in the water.

bakasana
CRANE

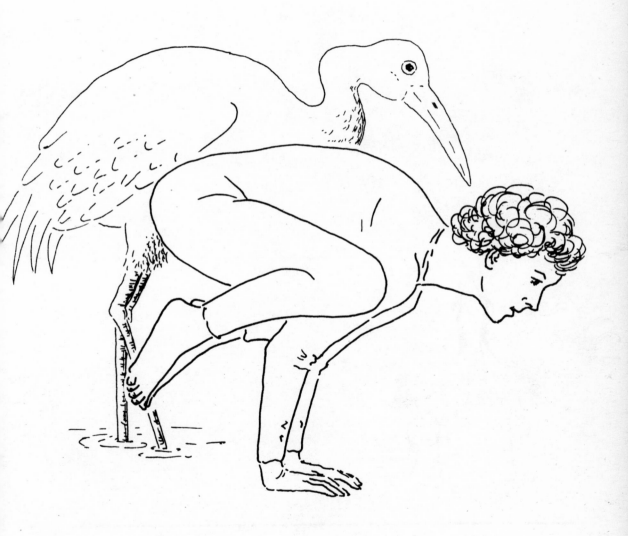

"Balance in space; go into the unknown: conquer fear."

B.K.S. Iyengar

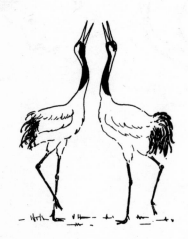

bakasana

CRANE

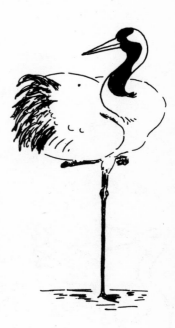

THE CRANE, A WATER bird with long legs and a large graceful body, in China symbolizes long life and happiness.[1] The movements of the crane, with its large slow-moving wings, look very elegant[2] and controlled; but it is quick in pursuing the fish and frogs that are its prey. One peculiar habit of this bird is sleeping while standing on one leg.

Some people thought the crane to be a messenger of the gods,[3] believing it to have the ability to commune with them and enter into higher states of consciousness. Quite contrary to this, the Celts believed the crane to be a form of the king of the underworld, a herald of death and war. The Christians chose to take the crane as symbolic for vigilance, loyalty, goodness, and also for the order within monasteries that would permit their long life. Like so many symbols, the crane represents both positive and negative aspects.

Although the crane often stands on one leg, in Bakasana the aspirant "stands" on two arms. During the initial attempts, these questions may come up: Do I have enough concentration to stand for any length of time on my hands? How can I keep my balance?

BAKASANA: Crane Posture

Long life, happiness, messenger of the gods, king of the underworld, herald of death, vigilance, loyalty, goodness; awkward, undignified, unsteady, my movements are not very elegant, I feel foolish

Strength and balance are needed to do this asana because a fall on the face could be painful. Do I have enough strength to reach the point of balance and vigilance? Can I find that point in my life? The eyes of the crane are round and appear to be very concentrated, not easily distracted, a picture of watchful patience. What are my distractions? What am I afraid of?

What is the water I am standing in—the imagination? the emotions? the unconscious? All the water birds seem to be an expression of the unconscious aspects of oneself, that is, parts to which the conscious mind has little access. There is also the desire to take flight, and the difficulties of spreading one's wings to come finally into full flight.

BAKASANA: Crane Posture

Strength, balance, concentration, distraction, watchful patience, imagination, emotions, conscious and unconscious, taking flight, spreading wings, full flight, birth and rebirth, destiny

Since the crane is a water bird, getting food from the water, which is symbolic of the emotions, we must think also of the feeding of those emotions. When the emotions are positive and directed, the cry of the crane can imply good fortune, but if they are out of control and negative, the cry will indicate bad fortune.

In India the crane, by its cry, makes known to other forms of life the good fortune or disaster that is about to befall them. Just so, the aspirant should make known to others, by preaching of the Dharma, how dreadful is purgatory—not having a chance for a long time, through another birth, to re-do, un-do, or improve one's destiny—and how blissful a state is Nirvana.

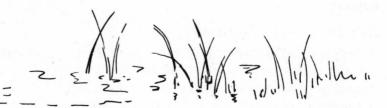

REFERENCE NOTES: Crane

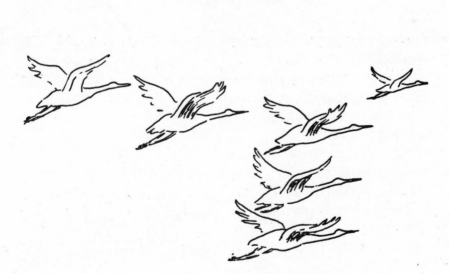

1. "In Eastern symbolism the crane and the pine tree, signifying long life, are often depicted together." *Encyclopedia of World Mythology,* 211.

2. This elegance of cranes is apparent in their mating dances. "Cranes dance, not hesitatingly but with all the aplomb of Scottish country dancers." They dance with circular movements: "To the ancients the ring dance associated the cranes with the sun. The cranes brought the spring and were surrogates of the resurgent sun god. Their dance epitomized both fertility and death rituals." Rowland, *Birds With Human Souls,* 31.

3. They were also associated with communication among people as they were believed to have influenced the invention of writing. Their flights in V-formation resemble the characters of early alphabets. Graves, *The White Goddess,* 242.

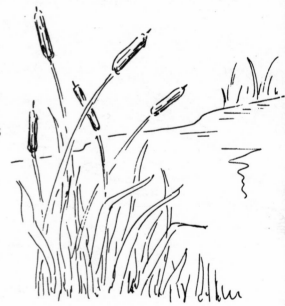

Hamsa means "swan." In this pose, the palms are on the floor with the thumbs touching, the hands facing forward. With elbows bent and supporting the diaphragm, the body is lifted up parallel to the floor.

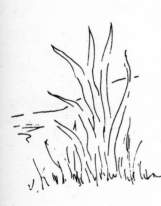

hamsasana
SWAN

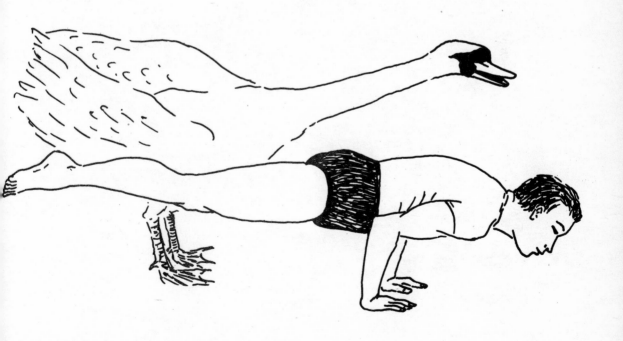

"The still waters of a lake reflect the beauty around it. When the mind is still, the beauty of the Self is reflected."
                                    B.K.S. Iyengar

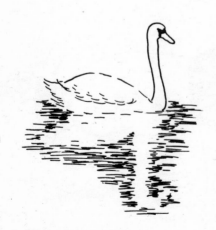

hamsasana

SWAN

THE SWAN IS SYMBOLIC for the combination of the two elements of air and water. It is the most majestic of birds, solar and beneficent, symbolizing life and the dawn of day. It is called the "bird of the poet," signifying solitude and retreat.

Rabindranath Tagore dedicated one of his poems to the swan:

> Tell me O Swan, your ancient tale.
> From what land do you come, O Swan?
> To what shore will you fly?
> Where would you take your rest, O Swan?
> And what is it that you seek?[1]

There are times when aspirants also need to retreat from their daily life into solitude to find what they seek.

The holiness that is attributed to the swan is shown in Deuteronomy 14:16 by the admonition that owls and swans must not be eaten. This bird also symbolized purity and grace for the Christians in Gaelic Scotland, where it served as a symbol of the Virgin Mary. Hamsasana is a difficult posture, and these qualities of the swan can only be attained with great effort and perseverance. As you attempt this posture, balancing on your hands, think of the efforts you must make in all areas of your life to attain purity and grace.

HAMSASANA: Swan Posture

Air and water, solitude and retreat, majestic, purity, grace, holiness, effort, perseverance; ungainly, feeling clumsy and awkward, my arms are weak, where is the majesty? or the grace?

The swan takes on many different aspects. In an ancient Germanic myth Freya, the goddess of love, was born of white sea foam and resembled a swan. In Roman mythology

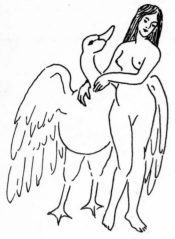

Orpheus the Musician is represented as a swan; and Jupiter sometimes takes this form so that he can visit his love, Leda, without the knowledge of his jealous wife, Juno. The swan is sacred to Aphrodite; both her golden chariot and that of Apollo were drawn by swans.[2]

Sometimes there is an interchange between the form of a swan, duck, or goose. In the East the magic power belonged originally to the goose; the five-headed Brahma, the creative aspect of God in India, rides on the Cosmic Gander. But in translating ancient spiritual texts of the East, the goose, because of its chatter, was exchanged for the swan with its quiet, majestic movements over the waters. Let this be a reminder for the aspirant that attention must be paid not only to the performance of the asana, but also to the chatter of the mind.

The majesty and magnificence of the swan is equalled only by the eagle, Garuda. The *Rig Veda* (IV: 40, 5) declares, "In the ether he is the swan (or goose) of the sun, in the air Vesu." The swan and goose are thus often symbolically interchangeable, and the swan is also replaced by the flamingo in some countries, as each culture uses the bird available in its surroundings for the symbolic meaning.

According to the Hindu theory of creation, it was the goose who laid the golden egg from which Brahma was born. The Egyptians considered the sun to be that golden egg, laid by the primeval goose. Perhaps this is the origin of the fairy tale of the goose that lays the golden eggs.

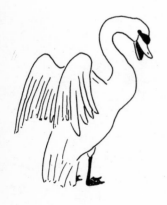

It is the geese in the *Dhammapada* that go on the path of the sun because of their magical power, and lead those who have achieved wisdom out of this world. Because of the goose's chatter, it was believed that language started with this bird. Refining the use of language and clarifying the meaning of words is an important part of the spiritual path. What is the personal meaning of these words to you?

HAMSASANA: Swan Posture

Goddess of love, sacred, quiet movements, magnificence, golden egg, chatter, magical power, language, Hamsa, breath and spirit, wisdom, time, calm mind, beautiful perceptions, two selves

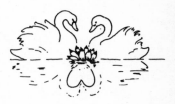

Two swans together are "that pair of swans who are Ham and Sa, dwelling in the mind of the Great, who subsist entirely on the honey of the blooming lotus of knowledge" *(Saundarya Lahari)*. The Hamsa bird "symbolizes the perfect union towards which the celestial beings fly."[3] Ham and Sa are the in-breathing and out-breathing, and so the swan represents breath and spirit. Sri Ramakrishna acknowledged that his wife, Sarada Devi, was equal to him spiritually by describing the two of them as a pair of swans.

Swans, symbolizing life and death, also mean wisdom and transition of time. Lohengrin crossed the sea of death in a boat drawn by swans when he left the Holy Grail, the kingdom of his father, to save the beautiful Elsa, and he was returned there by

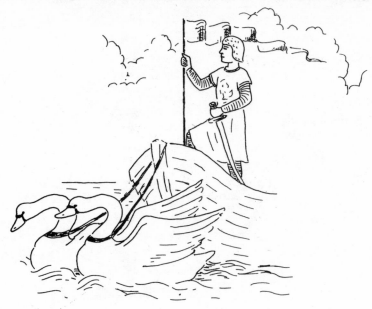

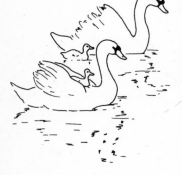

the swan when his secret was revealed. The mind is often portrayed as deep unfathomable water, and the swan, being such a kingly bird that glides gracefully on the waters, represents wisdom that, like the lotus, can float on the most murky waters without being dirtied. Swans need certain conditions to live and breed—calm waters, not the ocean or turbulent rivers. It is when the mind is calm that divine insights, beautiful perceptions, can sail on the lake of your mind. When you are able to hold this posture, watch your mind. Do you allow majestic thoughts to come in—beautiful thoughts as pure as a swan? Can you glide, unsullied by the muddy waters?

The swan's song is directed toward its mate, its other half, and the two come together in perfect unity. Are your two selves floating majestically on the lake of your mind in perfect harmony, like two halves in accord? Can you bring together the one swan—your physical earthly nature—with the other—your intangible spiritual nature? Can you let these two swans sail along the cosmic ocean of Consciousness? These are the thoughts to have in mind when doing this asana.

Brahma on the Cosmic Gander

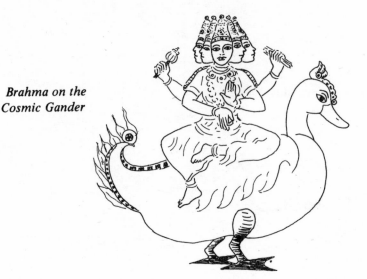

hamsasana

SWAN

1. Tagore, *One Hundred Songs of Kali,* 12.

2. The swan is also found as a vehicle in Indian mythology. Saraswati, the lovely Goddess of Wisdom and the Arts, rides a swan, symbolizing purity of mind. And *Paramahamsa* is a term of honor used to acknowledge a master yogi.

3. Cooper, *Illustrated Encyclopaedia of Traditional Symbols,* 164.

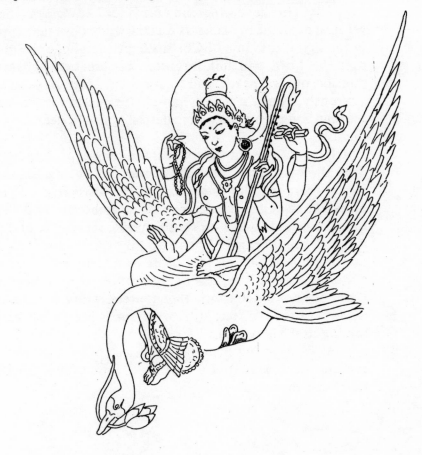

hamsasana

SWAN

REFLECTIONS: Birds

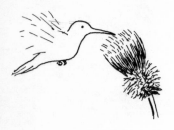

Who is not filled with admiration when seeing beautiful birds perched on trees or ledges of rock? There is the tiny, beautiful, little hummingbird, and the gold finch—there are many who have a lovely song that touches our hearts. In cold climates, where snow graces the branches of the trees, there are the chickadees, wee little birds with big hearts. They look cuddly because they are fluffy, with many extra down feathers to keep them warm. Some birds will even share shelter with human beings.

Thoughts have wings, and birds are like messengers.[1] The greatest of all the messengers was the white dove that appeared in the sky at the time of Christ's baptism, giving the message that the Lord had not forgotten his creation. That was a message of love, peace, and reassurance. Many of us still listen anxiously, even if it is with half-closed minds, for the message that can come from on high to descend into the heart and perch there.

If we truly listen we can hear the song of life and love; and if we allow it to echo throughout our whole being, then we can join in this song glorifying life and the Most High. There are birds like the chakori who live on moonbeams. Is it that we, too, are meant to live on those elusive, intangible and yet so mystical moonbeams? Where do they come from? We know that the moon has no light of its own. The moon is like the mind. The mind, too, has no light of its own. It receives the Light of knowledge from other sources, which it radiates like the rays of the sun. The light of the sun is life-giving, and so is the Light of knowledge.

All birds spend their days in search of food; so should an aspirant be in search of divine food, food that nourishes the heart and the mind.

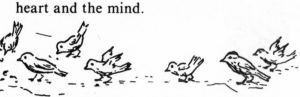

As the saying goes, "Birds of a feather flock together." The spiritual aspirant, too, will need others with the same goal for support and protection from destructive, persuasive influences. Not only monasteries and ashrams provide such shelter, but wherever there are three or four together, sharing a glimpse of the heart, they are strengthened in the search. Even the cave dwellers of old, in their self-chosen solitary confinement, from time to time needed to be with somebody of like mind.

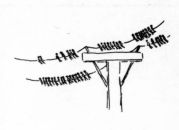

The large birds of prey—the falcon, the eagle—who soar so majestically, achieve this mastery in flight by surrendering to the currents of the air, with only a few movements of their wings. But however powerful, none of these birds can stay forever so far above the earth. They, too, have to find shelter. The high-flying mind in meditation has to return to the nitty-gritty of daily living, after taking the eagle's view of daily events that are so overwhelming when one is right down amongst them, and so insignificant when one is far above.

There is no bird that cannot give a message. The crane and the heron, with their long legs, stand in the water, their bodies above the surface, waiting patiently for their food which they have to grasp quickly when it comes along. It is a beautiful reminder for us that, while standing in the waters of emotions, with part of ourselves untouched, we must get hold of those inspirational feelings quickly before they dart beyond our reach.

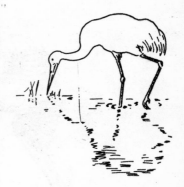

The phoenix, a beautiful mystical bird, as elusive as the great Garuda, too fast in flight to hold on to, too large to comprehend, arises from the ashes of sacrifice, the burnt ego.

Inspiring ideas are like eggs that need to be incubated to produce spiritual fledglings. The phoenix does not lay any eggs; it is reborn from its ashes. The mystical bird in us arises from the ashes of burnt ignorance and takes flight on the wings of wisdom. Like the sun, appearing again at its appropriate time, so the phoenix, the mystical bird of the sun, is born in us with the dawn.

1. "A great many symbols and significations to do with the spiritual life and, above all, with the power of intelligence are connected with the images of 'flight' and 'wings.' The 'flight' signifies intelligence, the understanding of secret things and metaphysical truths. 'Intelligence is the swiftest of birds,' says the Rg Veda (VI, 9, 5); and the Pancavimca Brahmananda (IV, 1, 13) states that 'he who understands has wings.' We can see how the archaic and exemplary image of 'flight' becomes charged with new meanings, discovered in the course of new awakenings of consciousness." Eliade, *Myths, Dreams and Mysteries,* 105.

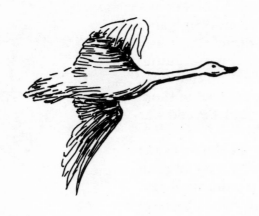

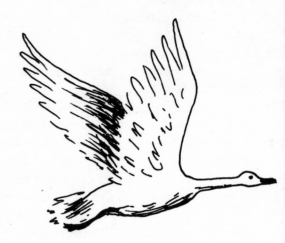

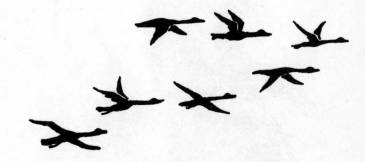

ANIMALS

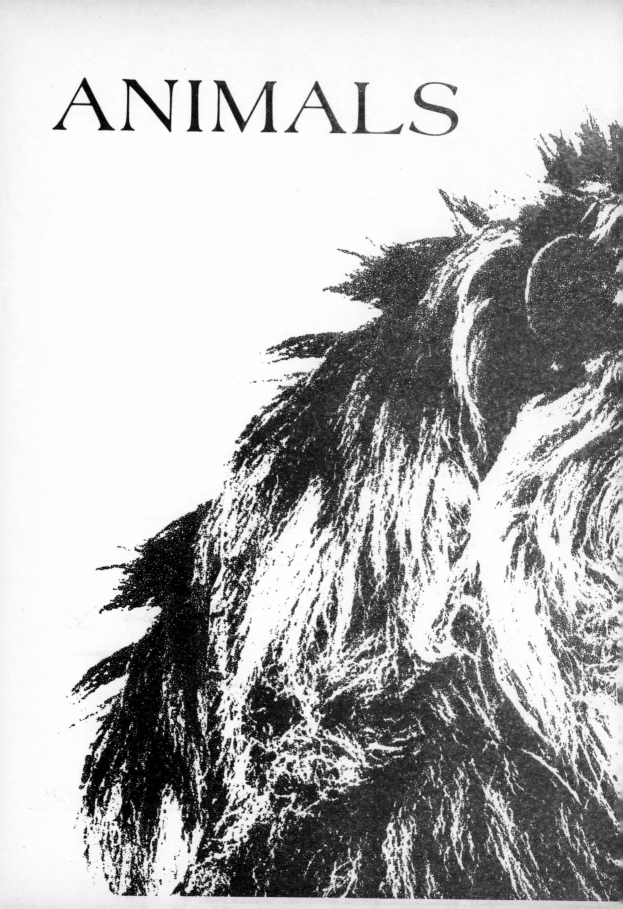

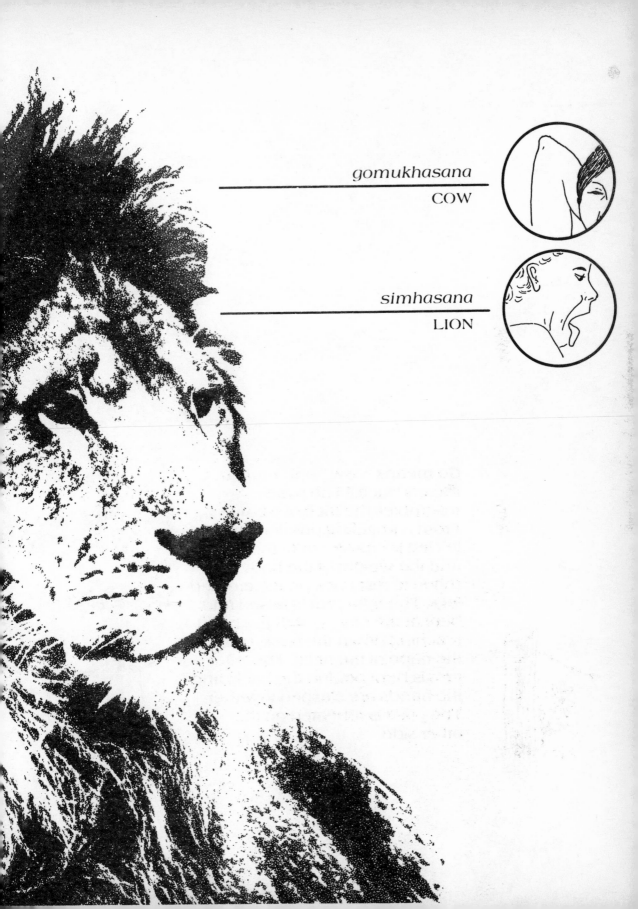

gomukhasana
COW

simhasana
LION

Go means "cow," and *mukha* means "face." The pose resembles the face of a cow. From a kneeling position, the left leg is crossed over the right, and the weight of the body is made to rest back on the crossed legs. The right arm is raised and bent at the elbow, with the hand reaching down the back, below the nape of the neck. The left arm is bent behind the back, and the hands are clasped together. The pose is repeated on the other side.

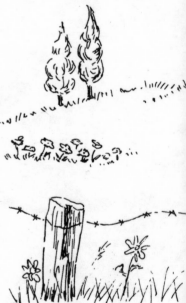

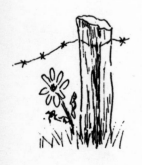

gomukhasana

COW·FACE

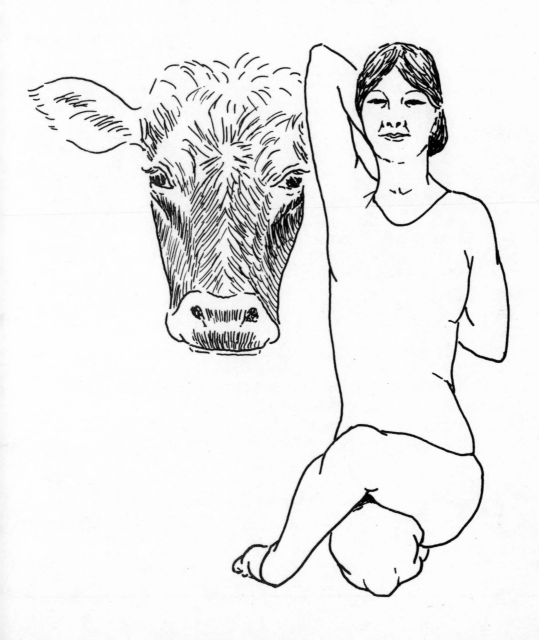

"Ears receptive, ears passive."
B.K.S. Iyengar

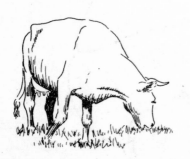

gomukhasana

COW-FACE

IN INDIA THE COW is a sacred animal. It is life-producing, gives milk and butter, and its dung is used for fire to cook. In some areas of India there is a ceremony in which a person of a lower caste can be elevated to a higher caste by being "born" from a large golden cow.[1] The Egyptians, who were very much tuned in to the spirit of the animals of their country, worshipped the cow goddess, the primeval female creative principle, who was sometimes shown with the body of a woman and the head of a cow.

Ramakrishna, the renowned Indian mystic and saint, compared aspirants to cows; some you have to get by the tail backward into the temple, while others find their way by themselves. It will be worthwhile for the aspirant to think of the symbolic meaning this common farmyard animal has had over the centuries.[2]

In the beginning of the practice of this asana there will be tension in the legs—in the ankles particularly. The shoulder blades will certainly loosen, and the hands clasped at the back will force the chest to open. It will be difficult to keep back, neck, and head straight, and there are some who will have a sense of irritation in the area of the stomach until they have become more proficient in the exercise.

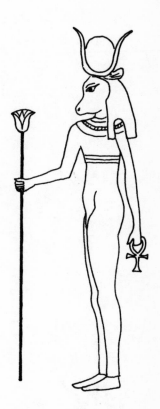

GOMUKHASANA: Cow-face Posture

Sacred, life-producing, milk and butter, dung, golden cow, goddess, female creative principle, by the tail, backward into the temple, tension, ankles, loosen the shoulder blades, open the chest, irritation, holding, clasping, forcing

A cow gives the impression of tremendous weight, strength, and muscle, without the grace of a thoroughbred horse, which may easily weigh as much as the cow but with

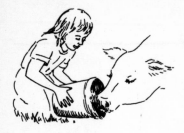

different proportions. And although a cow can have enormous strength a child can go up to her and give her a rub without any fear.

Strength is needed to do this difficult posture and a feeling of tranquility comes with its accomplishment. The sense of softness, almost docility, and at the same time the restriction of the asana, are quite remarkable and will trigger awareness of all sorts of weaknesses. Feelings of being like a stupid cow, or bull-headed, emerge, bringing uneasiness. I wish I could just lie in a field like a contented cow, chewing my cud.

A cow has four separate and distinct areas of digestion. She takes in a substantial amount of hay and roughage at one feeding and, after a period of time, regurgitates this coarse material and chews it into a softer, broken-down mass. This could be likened to the aspirant who must "chew" over again the spiritual information and instructions that are received, to be able to digest them and extract the nourishment.

For most people Gomukhasana does not relate to a cow's face, as the name would imply; but the cow is an animal with so many characteristics, which play such an important part in so many cultures, and the asana brings so many benefits, that it needs to be given a place.

In ancient times cattle were the wealth of kings, more important for defence than even armies. Such value was given

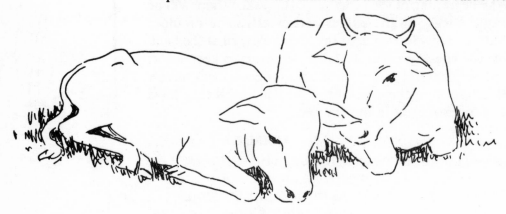

to them that a king could appease an angry neighbor with the gift of his daughter together with a few hundred cows. The importance of this animal is shown in the legends and proverbs of many countries. Angelo de Gubernatis has gathered a number of these stories illustrating the significance given to the nourishing qualities of the cow in relation to the sun, the moon, and the sky, and also the purity of that nourishment, because white milk comes from cows of any color, even red or black. He includes some humorous proverbs, such as the one about shutting the stable door after the cow has been stolen, or a cow that doesn't know what her tail is worth until she loses it.[3] Examples from other cultures of the meaning of a symbol show us that we are all one unit as a human race.

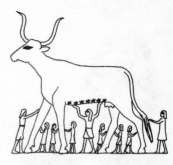

The Egyptian sky goddess, Nut, as the sacred cow

GOMUKHASANA: Cow-face Posture

Weight, strength, muscle, without grace, difficulty, tranquility, softness, docility, restriction, weaknesses, stupid cow, bull-headed, uneasiness, contentment, digestion, chew over, extract nourishment, benefits, wealth, sun, moon, sky, purity, shutting the stable door, losing her tail

The cow is sacred because it is an authentic symbol of motherhood, keeping creation alive. The creation of the human race has intrigued human minds everywhere. According to the Upanishads, Atman split into a man and a woman; she became a cow and he became a bull. They produced offspring which in turn became all the animals on earth.[4] And from this cow, mother of creation, comes the milk of Divine Wisdom which nourishes the aspirant on the spiritual path. Poetry is written in India of the clouds resembling cows, raining down nourishing milk and feeding especially those who seek the milk of Divine Wisdom for their inner nature, to transform the lower emotions into pure feelings.

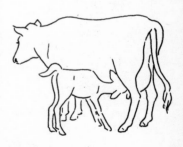

REFLECTIONS: Cow-face

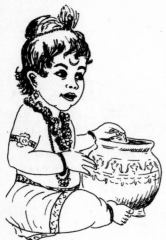

Lord Krishna, the divine cowherd, has given a most reassuring message to all of mankind. When he was a little boy, Gopal, (the name implying that he was the protector of cows), he was scolded by the gopis and by his mother, Yashoda. The complaint was that he was stealing the butter.

Many treatises have been written on how the Lord himself could be a butter thief, but do not humans take the honey from the bees, the kernels from the nuts, and the seeds from the grain? Every bite we eat is life in some form. If we are to be of service to the Most High, we must nourish our bodies, but take only what we really need. Lord Krishna gives the permission by doing so himself.

Nourishment is of many kinds. The body comes first because when one is hungry, cold, and homeless, there is no inclination for prayer and meditation, no sense of gratitude for even having a body. But when the body has been looked after, and when the heart is nourished by purified emotions, and the mind by divine thoughts, all nourishment becomes the milk of Divine Wisdom.

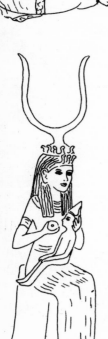

In the normal course of events, the nourishment for the newborn baby becomes immediately available. Those who have committed themselves to be Divine Mother's caretakers have the responsibility of having available the nourishment for the seekers when they are ready. That guidance can be received from the sacred texts of many different cultures; the four Vedas, for example, are related to the cow who stands on four legs,[5] ever ready to nourish the spiritual baby, providing at every stage of growth what is needed.

Isis-Hathor suckling Horus

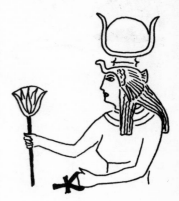

1. The Indian ceremony mentioned in this text has also been called the "lotus-womb gift." In both Indian and Egyptian traditions the cow has been associated with the lotus. In Egyptian mythology the cow goddess is sometimes depicted holding a lotus which "is supposed to represent the great world lotus flower, out of which rose the sun for the first time at creation." Frazer, *Folklore in the Old Testament*, 221.

2. This animal whose nourishment is taken for granted by so many in the West was certainly not taken for granted in ancient times. "The primordial flood as cow, or the cow as the first living creature rising from the primordial flood, is an authentic symbol of world-creating motherhood." The Egyptian cow goddesses water the earth with their rain-milk. Neumann, *The Great Mother*, 218.

    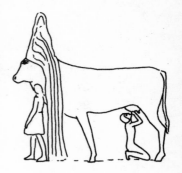

    There is a magic wishing-cow in the mythology of more than one culture. It can be found in Norse, Irish, Iranian, and Indian traditions. In India, "the magic wishing-cow is the earth milked of good and evil substances by gods and demons. She is churned out of the ocean of milk; and the ocean of milk, from which all else is churned forth, in turn flows from the udder of the wishing-cow. In almost all parts of Ireland the Milky Way is called 'the path of the white cow.'" "The magic wishing-cow is the image of the mother full of milk, a primary psychological symbol of goodness and love." O'Flaherty, *Women, Androgynes, and Other Mythical Beasts*, 241, 250.

3. Gubernatis follows the ancient mythologies from India through the Middle East, Greece, and Europe, illustrating the interconnectedness among what appear to be diverse cultures. See his *Zoological Mythology* for more on the cow.

4. *Brihadaranyaka Upanishad*, I, 4:1-4. In Germanic myth, the first creature on earth was Yamir and his first companion was a

gomukhasana   •**235**

COW-FACE

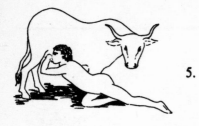

cow, a food-providing creature. "The cow takes pride of place among animals. She becomes the ancestor of all living creatures, the symbol of fecundity." *Larousse World Mythology,* 363.

5.   In the Indian tradition, there are four stages (yugas) of development on a universal scale: "In the first, the Cow of Virtue stands on four legs: men are perfectly virtuous and the laws of caste are kept. In the Treta Yuga, the Cow stands on three legs. In the Dvapara Yuga, she stands on two legs. And in the Kali Yuga . . . the cow stands on one leg. In that age, which is the one we are living in now, men have forgotten virtue almost entirely." "The breath of Brahma," retold by Paul Jordan-Smith, *Parabola,* 2(3):53, 1977.

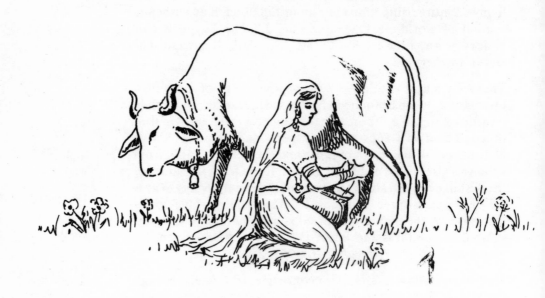

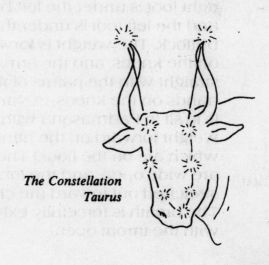

The Constellation
Taurus

COW·FACE

Simha means "lion": this pose resembles a lion roaring. The right foot is under the left buttock, and the left foot is under the right buttock. The weight is forward on the knees, and the arms are straight with the palms of the hands on the knees. (A variation is to sit in Padmasana with the weight forward on the hands which are on the floor.) The jaws are wide open, and the tongue stretched out toward the chin. The breath is forcefully exhaled with the throat open.

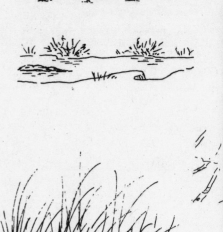

simhasana
LION

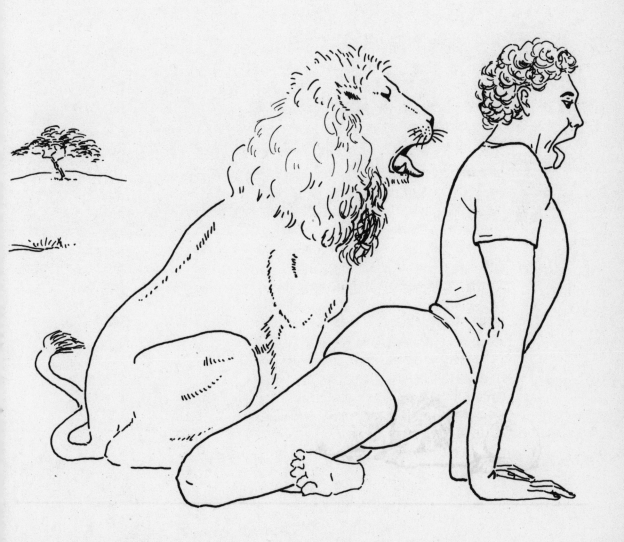

"If you do not surrender to your Guru, at least at the time of learning, surrender. If not, the ego is responsible for that pride."
B.K.S. Iyengar

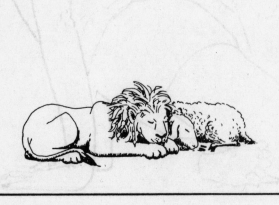

simhasana

LION

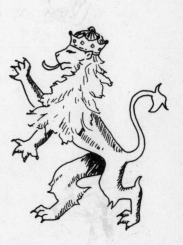

IN INDIA THE LION is the supreme symbol of royal strength and majesty; *lion of men* is an expression equivalent to "king," as the king is supposed to be the best of men. This symbol of the lion, who is "king of the beasts," was also developed in Greece, where the king was called "lion"; and other European royal families have used the lion in their heraldry as a sign of their strength. Fierce pride, too, is attributed to lions, and pride, of course, goes with royalty.

One of the most fascinating images of the lion is the sphinx of Gizeh, which was a symbol to the Egyptians for the sun god, Ra-Temu-Khepera-Herukhuti. No one knows when this extraordinary statue was built, but it was intended to provide a colossal abode for the spirit of the sun god, who was expected to protect the dead and their tombs.[1] It has a lion's body with a human head. Was the issue strength, because of the lion's powerful body? Or knowledge, because of the human head, capable of reasoning? There are many speculations, considered by some scholars to be just personal opinions, or worse, merely fantasies. However, it is by allowing symbol and metaphor to speak that one can come closer to understanding the meaning of the sphinx. The Greeks, too, had their sphinxes. They were winged, with heads and breasts of women.

In the countries of North Africa, particularly in Egypt, the lion has been a pet and, of course, a great protector. Undesirable persons would be kept at a respectful distance by the presence of the pet lion. Today the game wardens of Africa say "a visible lion is not dangerous" but the hidden one, camouflaged by the grasses, stones, and sand, may attempt a surprise attack.

This posture can help one to know the power within oneself, how it is camouflaged or masked, and the danger that arises from pretending to be a lamb, while a ferocious lion is

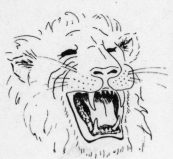

roaring inside. Few people can be truly gentle. Some people, when they caress a baby or a small animal, clench other parts of the body, such as the teeth, to redirect the energy from the hand that would otherwise turn into a heavy weapon. Parents are powerful gods to their children, and often have to hide their power to form a mutual relationship. The expression of power can be very subtle.

Simhasana is the only asana in which a sound is made. In the roar of the lion, ferocity and strength are given expression, and the lungs and throat are cleared of all the choked-back words and tears that many people hold unexpressed.

SIMHASANA: Lion Posture

*Royal, majesty, king of beasts, pride, sphinx,
sun god, knowledge, strength, winged, protector,
undesirable persons, visible, camouflaged,
surprise attack, masked, lamb, gentle, ferocious,
clench, heavy weapon, power, subtle, roar,
choked-back words, tears, unexpressed*

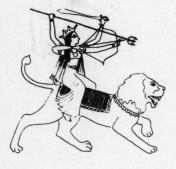

Life and destiny seem to exercise a power that is beyond one's control most of the time. Symbolizing that power in the East, Divine Mother in her aspect of Durga is described as riding on a lion.[2] She is the only goddess who does not have a male consort. (Parvati has Shiva, Radha has Krishna. . . .)Kali, an aspect of Durga, is so powerful that she will challenge any power; she has not found her equal. In her aspect of Kali, Divine Mother gives birth to new life and destroys the old, this destruction being symbolic for her all-consuming power.

Thrones in the Orient are often built with a lion serving as the back of the seat, its paws forming the legs. The Buddha's throne was called a "lion's throne." As Siddhartha, he was born to a royal family whose ensign was the lion. When he became the Buddha, he was called "the omniscient lion of the Sakyas." In the Old World, furniture that is hand-carved, ornamented with lions' heads and paws, conveys opulence and power and sets a tone of command.

When the word *lion* is said, one person may think of Africa, lakes, heat, brush country; others may see in their mind's eye a lion attacking someone, killing. Many who have read *Born Free* and *Living Free,* the story of the lioness Elsa and her cubs, may have a very special feeling for the lion as an animal of great strength and agility. But we may also remember Joy Adamson recounting that when the lioness was very tense and nervous, it would come and suck on her thumb. It is hard to believe that this most powerful animal, with no natural enemies, can be so much in need of comfort.

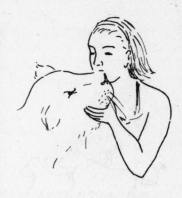

According to our perceptions, ruthlessness, ferocity, and courage are the characteristics of the lion. Yet it will never attack straight on, but rather come from behind. The lion will chase an animal, and jump on it to crush it, then dig in its claws for the kill.

Nature is hard on all of us. In many areas we often have to fight like lions for our existence, to survive. In the darkest moments of life, it can feel as if one is being thrown to the lions to be devoured as were the early Christians.

People in business or on Wall Street show a ferocity that is like that of a savage lion; but they must also be lionhearted to have the courage to take risks. We speak of wealthy people as getting the "lion's share," the major part. Life is literally almost handed to them on a platter; and yet their numbers are so few in comparison with the total population that we can't even talk of one percent. But they, too, have no guarantee that what is handed to them will remain with them. What has not been worked for, what has not been deserved, is often carelessly lost, sometimes even thrown away. Most of us have to learn the hard way, right from the beginning, working for whatever we get.

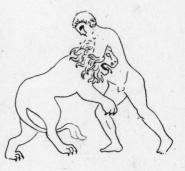

The lion is the king of beasts. It would seem that an animal of this kind leads an easy life; he doesn't need to work much, does he? The male lion certainly does not. It is the female lion who hunts, but the male eats first; then she eats, and what is left goes to the cubs. This does not show great concern for the offspring. The instincts of the cubs, however, seem to tell them what to do. But if the cubs try to push their way in to the food when they are hungry, they get a heavy whack to put them in their place—a whack that sometimes even kills them. On the other hand, the female lions of a pride share in the nursing duties. Even in the mating ritual it is the lioness who gives the signal, and the male then responds.

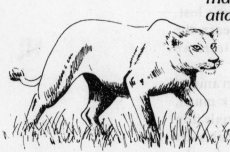

These big cats resemble house cats in their way of walking and their hunting instincts. Both can draw in their claws so they can move faster, then put them out to catch their prey. Cats have their own character, their own will, and they are very hard to train. Lion tamers observe the cats when they are young and make careful choices, or use old lions that are happy to be fed and not hunt any more.

The lion posture shows some important human characteristics. Movements can be cat-like—sinuous and stealthy. Psychologically, a person can be willful or catty, attacking from behind. And yet the power and the intelligence of a lion are also available.

Ponder these thoughts as you practice this asana.

SIMHASANA: Lion Posture

Divine Mother, Durga, Kali, birth and destruction, Buddha's throne, Africa, attacking, killing, agility, tense, nervous, suck on her thumb, ruthlessness, courage, survival, devoured, savage, lionhearted, lion's share, hunting, take life easy, instincts, mating ritual, signal, will, sinuous, stealthy, catty, attacking from behind

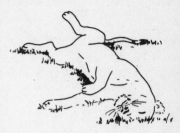

Lions, for all their strength, have their limitations. They run in short spurts, and any animal that is a fast long-distance runner would be able to shake a lion off. In order to regain their strength, lions take a lot of time to rest. In fact, unless they are hunting, they are resting or sleeping. Research on lions shows that it is not impossible for their prey to defend themselves.[3] An animal with hoofs can strike the jaw of the lioness and break it, and she will die of starvation: she can't eat, she can't hunt, she is finished, and her prey goes free. When in a strong position in life, it is tempting to rely on power; but like all things, nothing remains forever—everything changes. It seems that we must be constantly on the alert to meet any situation.

Simha means "lion," and the asana is dedicated to Narasimha, the man-lion incarnation of Vishnu. In the Christian iconography the evangelist Mark is presented as a winged lion with a halo, sitting on a book. This indicates all the powers that one can think of possibly acquiring, the halo being the holiness and the lion itself being the great power, resting on the book of wisdom. That book has a message that is as powerful as a lion; but it is also holy, and can move on a pair of wings.

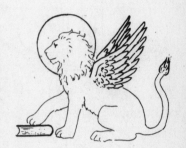

All these things tell us something about our own past. We have inherited that past, and we may think that there is no memory left; but if we let those thoughts arise from the unconscious we may be surprised at what comes up.

REFLECTIONS: Lion

The lion is, unquestionably, a powerful symbol. A fascinating statue was found in Ostia, where it was dedicated by Heracles and his sons in A.D. 190. This Mithraic Kronos statue shows a man, completely naked, with a lion's head. He is

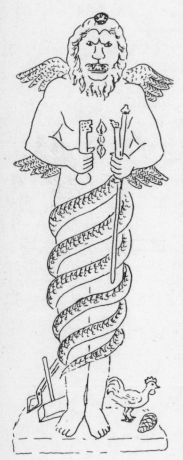

endowed with all the powers one can imagine. On the base of the statue are a cock, a pine cone, a hammer, and a pair of tongs. His body is wound six times around with a snake whose head is resting like a crown on the lion's head. This incredible figure also has two pairs of wings, and holds two keys and a scepter. A thunderbolt is engraved on the breast.[4]

Little is known about this statue, but its symbolism is certainly very intriguing. A list of these symbols and their universal meanings alone is fascinating. Since ancient times the great power of the lion has been linked to royalty, and it is tempting to interpret the six circles of the snake as the serpent of the Kundalini, particularly since the head of the snake rests on the lion-man's head. Wisdom of the highest kind can be anticipated in this interpretation. This is surely not an exaggeration, given the presence of four wings. A creature that has wings can move beyond the earth. Powerful thoughts have wings. And this double pair can even suggest the power of bi-location.

The reinforcement for such speculation comes from the key and the scepter, both symbols of authority, as well as the thunderbolt on the breast. Except for the pine cone, the hammer, and the pair of tongs, all the other symbols support this idea.

The pine cone carries seeds for the multiplication of the pine tree, as well as food for small animals. The hammer: to hammer away at a particular point, to drive something home, to understand, to hold things together. With a pair of tongs one can pick up burning wood or coal, move it, and yet not get burned oneself. This might imply that smouldering fires are dangerous and need to be removed. An individual endowed with this much power will also attract opposite forces, as darkness is the opposite of light.

This image tells us to be as wise as a serpent, as powerful as a lion, as practical as hammer and tongs, as watchful as a cock, and to use the key of knowledge to establish authority—yet to move on wings and sail with destiny like a bird with the currents of the wind. East and West seem to come together in this statue to give a message to those who have an inkling that their potential could be fulfilled by wise action, and the obstacles removed like a smoking ember; that the seeds of wisdom are available to anyone who looks for them, and that knowledge might be offered by a teacher in proportion to the sincerity of the seeker. The lion is the symbol of the sun, and the sun in turn is the symbol of the highest wisdom, of consciousness beyond all expectation, leading to the Light that is innate in that wisdom, and thereby representing a great power, like an atom that is freed from encumbrances.

For the aspirant, the lion posture can be symbolic for gaining sovereignity over all the natures within, as the lion itself is ruler over all the beasts.[5] Then, if words of wisdom are heard, they resonate within like a lion's roar,[6] awakening the sleepwalker. Keep the gaze on the Light—the darkness of ignorance is overpowered by the Light.

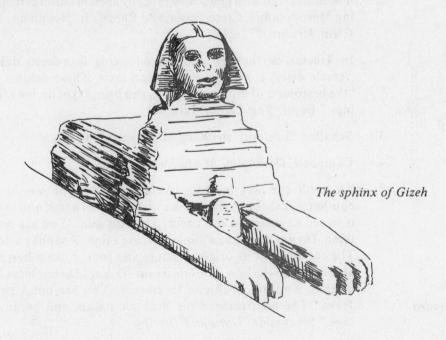

The sphinx of Gizeh

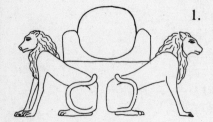

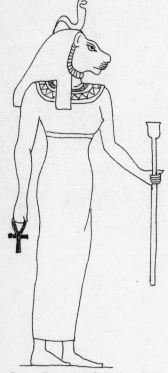

*Bast, Egyptian lion-headed
goddess*

1. "One of the oldest known Lion-gods is Aker, who was supposed to guard the gate of the dawn through which the Sun-god passed each morning. . . . In later days the Egyptian mythologists believed that during the night the sun passed through a kind of tunnel which existed in the earth, and that his disappearance therein caused the night, and his emerging therefrom caused the day; each end of this tunnel was guarded by a Lion-god, and the two gods were called Akeru. In the Theban Recension of the *Book of the Dead* we find the Akeru gods represented by two lions which are seated back to back, and support between them the horizon with the sun's disk on it; in the later theology they are called Sef and Tuau, i.e., 'Yesterday' and 'To-day' respectively." Budge, *Gods of the Egyptians*, vol. 2, 360-361.

2. The lion is seen with goddesses in many ancient cultures including Mesopotamia, Crete, Syria, and Phoenicia. Neumann, *The Great Mother*, 272-273.

   In Tibetan mythology, the fierce-looking lion-faced dakini (female deity) is guardian of hidden texts. These dakinis are "the bestowers of mystic doctrines and bringers of divine offerings." Beyer, *The Cult of Tara*, 46.

3. Schaller, "Life with the King of Beasts," 504.

4. Campbell, *Occidental Mythology*, 265-266.

5. "A lion's cub was bleating like a lamb when it was in the company of sheep. A lion took it to the side of a well and asked it to see its image in the water. The lion said, 'You are not a lamb. Do not bleat like a lamb. You are a lion. Roar like a lion.' The cub realised its original nature and roared like a lion and accompanied the lion. The Guru said, 'O man! Do not bleat like a lamb. You are Brahman in essence. You are not a small Jeeva.' The man realised his Brahmic nature and became a sage." Sivananda, *Guru and Disciple*, 59.

6. "Lord, when all the defilements and secondary defilements are eliminated, one obtains the inconceivable Buddha natures exceeding the sands of the Ganges River. Then . . . one gains the unhindered understanding of all natures; is omniscient and all seeing, free from all faults and possessed of all merits; King of the Doctrine and Lord of the Doctrine; and, having gone to the stage which is sovereign over all natures, utters the lion's roar: 'My births are finished; the pure life fully resorted to; duty is done; there is nothing to be known beyond this.' " Wayman, *The Lion's Roar of Queen Srimala*, 89.

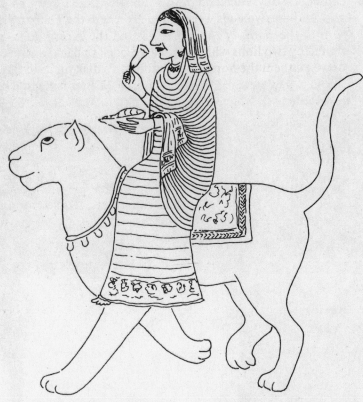

The East Indian goddess, Parvati, rides the lion.

SHAVASANA

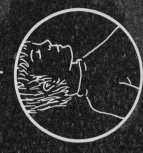

shavasana

CORPSE

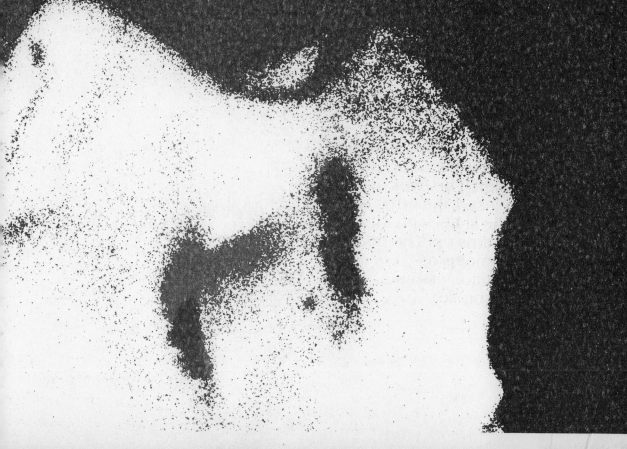

Shava means "corpse." In this pose, the body lies on the floor face-up and completely relaxed, while the mind is alert. The eyes are closed, the arms at the sides with the palms up. The body remains as motionless as a corpse.

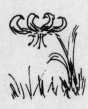

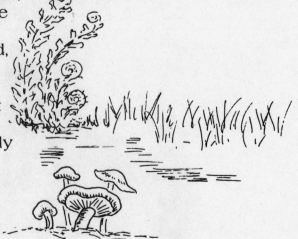

shavasana

CORPSE

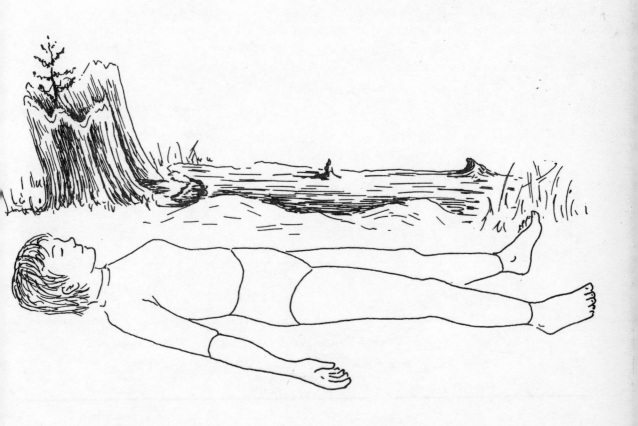

"The best sign of a good Savasana is a feeling of deep peace and pure bliss. Savasana is a watchful surrendering of the ego. Forgetting oneself, one discovers oneself."

B.K.S. Iyengar

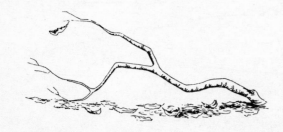

shavasana

CORPSE

By THIS POINT, the aspirant will have recognized from the practice of the asanas what an important part is played by dependence, interdependence, and interaction. Dependence and attachment are two of the great obstacles to freedom. And yet, at no time is there complete independence; there is interdependence between myself and other people, and between the inner and the outer world. In the process of awareness these interactions become very obvious. Self-analysis can redeem one from self-inflicted pain.

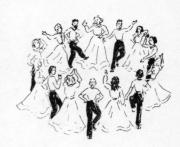

Particularly those asanas that are named after animals show that at no time is a human being disconnected from creation. There is no "lower" animal kingdom, or a "higher" human one, but each one of us is past, present, and future, all at once. The symbolic meaning of animals is widely reflected in mythological beliefs in many parts of the world. All of the symbolic images are pregnant with power over our lives, and by encountering them we are facing the great unknown, an interaction of all these many aspects we did not know were there.

Shavasana, the death pose, brings up the same questions that have been encountered before, through which we discover the most threatening thoughts that are roaming the murky waters of the mind. We are too frightened to let them surface, but surface they will, at a time when the thought of death is the least welcome. The stunning insights that have already emerged through the practice of other asanas will help us to face the idea of death courageously. The reality of death has been experienced when somebody we know has died, or is close to death. Then dependence on a healthy body and mind takes on much greater significance than ever before.

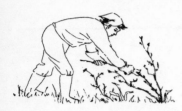

The influence of this asana on the body and the mind—from relaxation, to surrender, to death, and even after death—is incredible. If you do not want to be a living corpse, then the purpose of life has to be established. If you want to be an active participant in your life and not a parasite, then the dynamic interdependence between life and death has to be recognized, and the two have to meet in directed and concentrated interaction.

How long has anybody to live? Who knows? What about life that has not yet been lived? What appreciation is there for life and what it has to offer? Is death the great and grim reaper? Or the reliever of pain? Is death the end of all? Is there more than one life? Is death a time of rest between lives, like the night between days?[1]

In the quietness of meditation, with eyes closed to shut off all impulses, we open ourselves to the inner forces that give us renewed strength and inspiration to continue on the Path. But the greater spells of rest and darkness experienced in death are

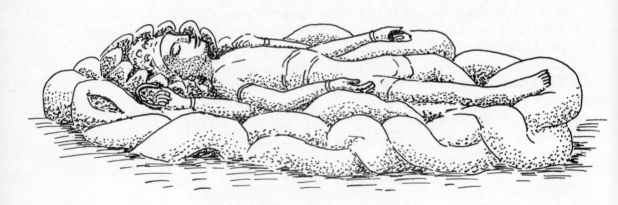

The East Indian god, Vishnu, sleeps on the Serpent Ananta who floats on the primordial waters. Vishnu's awakening brings about creation.

shavasana

CORPSE

needed to find the purpose for a new life, to make a dedication of the spirit that wants to be born again and take up the duty not yet fulfilled. What could that duty be?—the choice to cooperate with the course of our own evolution, the evolution of intelligence and consciousness that is the purpose of all human beings.

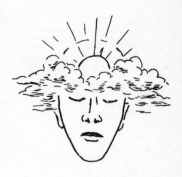

Intelligence is perhaps the most intriguing quality of the mind in its aspect of skillful interpreter. Of all the life experiences that have taken place, which were accepted by the mind? Which rejected or misconstrued? Are all experiences flooded by emotional impulses? The mind struggles with its own characteristics, sometimes being ambiguous, then clever or evasive. The mind can censor or concretize, yet it always interprets to its best advantage. In each life some lessons are learned and others are avoided or not even recognized. Forgetfulness is one of the mind's most convenient characteristics.

SHAVASANA: Corpse Posture

"Lower" animal kingdom, "higher" human one, great unknown, threatening, frightening, healthy, relaxation, surrender, after death, living corpse, active participant, parasite, grim reaper, reliever of pain, more than one life, meditation, renewal, purpose of life, duty unfulfilled, evolution of consciousness and intelligence, ambiguous, clever, evasive, censor, concretize, forgetfulness

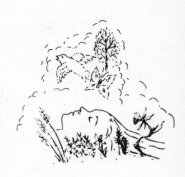

Of course, we all know that a dead body no longer resists. All our lives we use incredible amounts of energy to put up resistance. Even in sleep the resistance continues as dreams mirror back that activity. Shavasana gives the experience of a symbolic death and points to the need to be born anew.

We all have to die someday; who needs to be told this frightening truth? We know we are destined for this transition. We are fearful of it, and yet we toy with life and death as if it were not our concern. We prefer not to remember the skull in the Devi's hand in the Muladhara Chakra, telling us clearly the need for death of old mental-emotional concepts and parasitic thoughts—all that "stuff" that we ought to get rid of. What would happen if we were to stop the mind's deadly games that kill the goodness in us, the best of our qualities—loyalty, ethics, honesty? Would we decide to put to death all the interfering personality aspects that masquerade, deceive, and

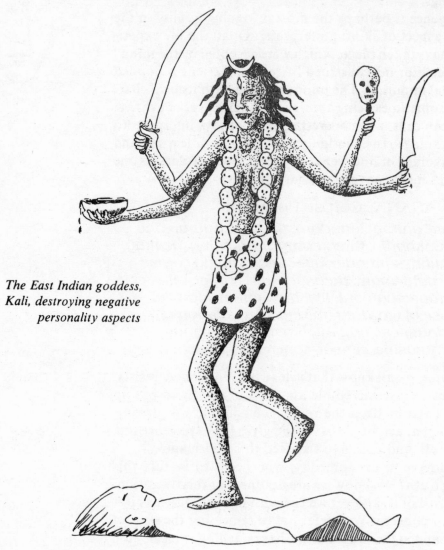

The East Indian goddess, Kali, destroying negative personality aspects

shavasana

CORPSE

mislead? Is it possible to imagine such a life, free of those old programs of the mind? If the answer is "no," then we should not be surprised that fear is the overriding thought about death.

Life is full of deadly games. Deadly games are the parasites that sap the life force, delude with promised security. Deadly games reveal the desire to kill. It has its beginning in competition:

Competition means to win.
To win means to fight.
To fight means to kill.
To kill means to win.

How many faces does death have? Consider death as:

a cultural idea
a last act of honor
avoidance of dishonor
an act to reinstate honor
a moral code of duty
being more important than life
going down with the ship
Am I the captain of my ship—of life and death?

Throughout life, small but significant warnings appear which are usually disregarded. Loss of physical strength, of sight and hearing, and stiffness in some limbs of the body remind us of our mortality. How are we using the time that remains? If we could only overcome the most merciless master, the ego, life would be dynamic.[2] That is what Saint Paul meant when he said, "Daily I die." After the demands of ego and its greed are surrendered, the struggle for fulfillment of personal desires lessens; life takes on a new zest like a breath of fresh air. One emerges—as from the shell of the tortoise or the sting of the scorpion—a new person who knows where to stand in life: Tadasana.

In Shavasana, relaxation is the first attempt to surrender, to let go. As the mind follows the flow of the breath, the ripples

CORPSE

of the mental lake slowly subside. With continued practice, the senses are gradually withdrawn and become still. Passion, egocentricity, self-importance, are, for the moment, put to rest. Rest becomes an important word whose meaning expands with experience. Shavasana, the corpse posture, gives a new understanding of death, of the need for surrender. The body at rest can do its repair work. Sufficient rest allows the body to recuperate from the driving forces of the emotions and the ambitions of the mind. The benefits—physically, mentally, emotionally—are profound. In that state of peace and quiet and inner harmony, one can perceive a vision of the Light that is present in both life and death.

I am created by Divine Light
I am sustained by Divine Light
I am protected by Divine Light
I am surrounded by Divine Light
I am ever growing into Divine Light[3]

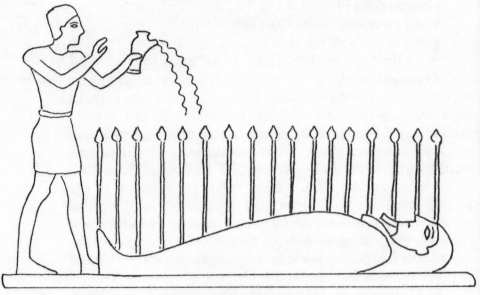

Death and rebirth: the mummy of the Egyptian god, Osiris, grows grain.

1. "Death is the temporary end of a temporary phenomenon. **By** death is meant the extinction of psychic life, heat, and consciousness of one individual in a particular existence. **Death is** not the complete annihilation of a being. Death in one **place** means the birth in another place, just as in conventional terms, the rising of the sun in one place means the setting of the sun in another place." Narada, *The Manual of Abhidhamma,* 51.

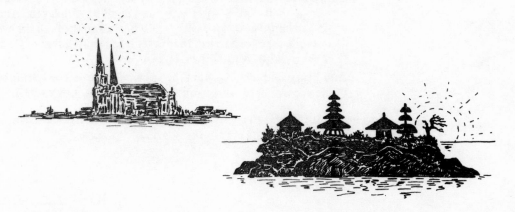

2. Surrender is an essential action for anyone who wishes to **lead a** spiritual life, as can be seen in the writings of **many great** spiritual teachers:

    > Whatever thou doest, whatever thou eatest, whatever thou offerest in sacrifice, whatever thou givest, whatever thou practiseth as austerity, O Arjuna, do it as an offering unto Me. (*Bhagavad Gita,* 9:27.)

    > Fix thy mind on Me; be devoted to Me; sacrifice unto Me; bow down to Me; having thus united thy whole self to Me, taking Me as the supreme goal, thou shalt come unto Me. (*Bhagavad Gita,* 9:34.)

    > Learn how to obey. Then alone you can command. (Sivananda, *Guru and Disciple,* 24.)

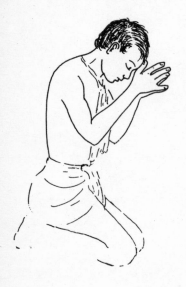

The Light of grace shines in the mirror of the mind which is rendered pure through faith, devotion and surrender. (Ibid., 222.)

Self-surrender means giving up of the ego-sense. Until the ego-sense is completely eliminated, we cannot realize God. Ego-sense is a screen between us and God. If you remove the screen you know you are He. (Ramdas, *World is God,*77.)

He who unreservedly surrenders himself to Me with devotion, is endowed with all the requisites necessary for Self-Realization. (*Tripura Rahasya,* 182.)

Jesus said unto him, If thou wilt be perfect go and sell that thou hast and give to the poor, and thou shalt have treasure in heaven; and come and follow me. But when the young man heard that saying, he went away sorrowful; for he had great possessions. Then Jesus said unto his disciples, Verily I say unto you, that a rich man shall hardly enter into the kingdom of heaven. And again I say unto you, it is easier for a camel to go through the eye of a needle, than for a rich man to enter into the kingdom of God. (*The Holy Bible,* Matthew 19:21-24.)

And Mary said, Behold, I am the handmaid of the Lord; let it be to me according to your word. (*The Holy Bible,* Luke 1:38.)

3. The Mantra of the Divine Light Invocation. See Swami Sivananda Radha, *The Divine Light Invocation.*

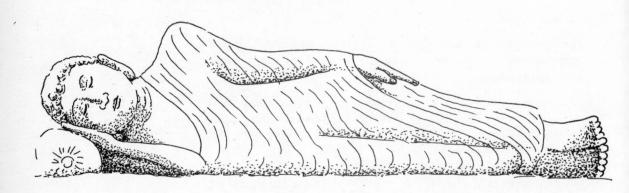

Eleventh century carving of the Parinirvana of the Buddha

shavasana

CORPSE

Osiris, Egyptian god of creation and regeneration, lies in his sarcophagus around which grows a magnificent tree. This tree was made into a column for the king's palace, and so symbolizes victory over death through resurrection.

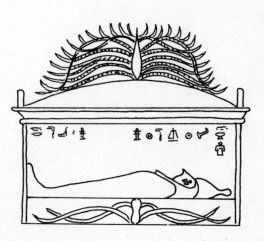

shavasana

CORPSE

brahmacharya
CELIBACY

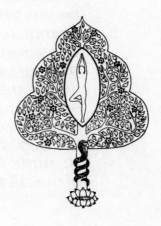

"Attracted to a life of pleasure, the individual begins to believe that such pleasures are eternal, whereas in fact they are merely transitory. Caught in the giddy whirl of pleasures, he is blinded and fails to see this. A discriminating person, however, sees through the ephemeral veil of sensory pleasures and learns to channel the outgoing energy of the senses inwards. He turns that energy back to the shrine of the Divinity, the Soul."

B.K.S. Iyengar

brahmacharya

CELIBACY

I<small>N</small> *Kundalini: Yoga for the West,* it was stated that Hatha Yoga was such an important part of the Kundalini system that it needed its own specific treatment. The philosophy of Brahmacharya was introduced in that book, and now it is possible to show the importance of Hatha Yoga in helping an aspirant who has chosen the path of celibacy.

The various commentaries in the ancient texts emphasize that Lord Shiva is able to create only when he is united with his consort, Shakti. This concept has been carried into the human condition. There is a wide difference between Cosmic Energy (Shiva) and its manifestation (our world and the various galaxies) and an ordinary man and woman entering into the act of procreation to continue the human species. Some people will have children with a definite purpose and an awareness of the responsibilities involved; but some will have children without much thought of later implications. Similarly, some enter the path of Yoga for improving general health or to enhance their relationships, others to develop their potential of which they have now become aware.

When the purpose is to become a being of a higher order, which means continuously increasing awareness, the methods to achieve this goal have to be clarified. Meritorious karma in this and previous births will give one a tendency, or rather a deep desire, to attain that union of Shiva and Shakti within. The male aspects of logic, reason, and action, and the female aspects of intuition, emotion, receptivity, and endurance, have to become likewise unified within each yogi or yogini. B.K.S. Iyengar has stated that to become an accomplished hatha yogi is more difficult than to earn a Ph.D. in any of the other sciences.

The householder years of an aspirant can be seen as the battlefield of the Gita. All the personality aspects and their ramifications incite the battles. When the duties as a householder have been discharged, the children have grown up and are on their own, then the life structure can be changed. In later life there also comes a declining interest in sex as other ideas become more worthwhile to pursue; the time has arrived when one can work toward the realization of one's potential. All the efforts that were needed to dispense the duties of a householder are now available to pursue the goal of Higher Consciousness. Self-mastery—the process of attaining Liberation—begins,,of course, in daily living, in freeing oneself from attachments, desires, greed, passions, whether one has a family or is single. Responsibilities have to be assumed whatever one's place in life, and these responsibilities should be discharged with the greatest care and the highest quality of which one is capable.

There are various schools of thought that emphasize that Brahmacharya or celibacy is not necessary for the attainment of Liberation; however, I would like to point out that such statements have usually been made by the men who are accustomed to looking at women as subordinates. Some have walked away from the consequences of their actions, and left the responsibility of possible offspring to the women. In the traditional relationship between a man and a woman it is not customary for her to be independent economically or emotionally. But the suffering of any dependent when one partner shuns responsibility, even for the sake of holiness, can hardly be considered a blessing. Yoginis have seldom written down their teachings, nor have their students, so we have few records of the female viewpoint.

Traditions are of different kinds in different cultures. We can follow the Eastern philosophy and its application, but to follow the culture may not be possible or even necessary. In the Western culture, traditions are not of such long standing; and in a new world, they are constantly in a state of flux. The fast and vast development of technology and science makes it difficult for anyone to plan a life and career, even within a twenty year span. But ideals and ethics have a common denominator, even though individuals will have to establish their own standards. For the aspirant, it is especially important to look at concepts of sex and love.

BRAHMACHARYA: Celibacy

For some, marriage and sex are a sacred duty.
Or . . . sex is sin, instinct, procreation, pleasure;
all sexual impulses are commanded
by the genes.
(See Kundalini: Yoga for the West *for further*
thoughts on Brahmacharya.)

Gandhi's autobiography shows the development in the relationship between a husband and wife—Mahatma Gandhi and Kasturbai—and brings to the foreground thoughts about Brahmacharya. In general it is presumed that only Christian monks and nuns observe celibacy; but the convictions of many people and their attitudes toward sex, gathered by Gabriella Brown, Ph.D., in her book, *The New Celibacy: How To Take a Vacation From Sex—And Enjoy It !,* may come as a surprise and show that celibacy is not so unusual. Couples may, from time to time, decide on a few weeks or even a few months to practice celibacy, just to break habitual activities and to renew and replenish their attractiveness to each other.

Examples are all around us of the need for time for recuperation after expenditure of energy. In nature, the farmer will give rest to a field on which he has grown crops. Religious tradition has allowed for a seventh day of rest. Such a time for rest and recuperation, even between births, is often not available to a woman.

Attitudes toward sex and celibacy today are affected by many things, including the imbalance between the number of men and women seeking partners for marriage—there are more women than men in most countries—and by the high divorce rate. Power groups—religious, business, military, or medical—also will advocate or oppose celibacy for their own advantage. Professor Geoffrey Parrinder, in *Sex in World Religions,* states that attitudes toward sex can be compared to today's world changes. Nevertheless, in *Sexual Energy and Yoga,* Elisabeth Haich investigates the possibility of using sexual energy for the purposes of spiritual development. Shankaracharya, an Indian sage considered by some the architect of the Kundalini system, put the emphasis on the creative forces of sex in the Muladhara, the first chakra, and implied redirecting the energy in the third, or Manipura Chakra, for different purposes. There can be no general direction in regard to sex or Brahmacharya; the implications are too far-reaching and contradictory.

How, then, is the decision for or against Brahmacharya to be made? There are different temperaments, different strong driving forces. Some people have little sexual desire and find it easy to control; others, who live a very active sex life, may find it hard to turn off the desire for gratification. These decisions have to be made by individuals themselves.

To understand the complexity of sexual interaction and how sex can be a tool of power used by a man or a woman to dominate the other, a process of self-investigation is necessary.

BRAHMACHARYA: Celibacy

*Tenderness mistaken as an invitation for sexual
    activity*
*Women with poor self-image using sex to
    achieve a stronger image*
Strong feelings of sex foolishly mistaken for love
Love versus eroticism
Sex and emotions
*What are my conceptions/misconceptions about
    sex?*

With the practice of Yoga, particularly if the spiritual levels are to be incorporated, the transpersonal psychological steps are only a preparatory stage, which is followed by a change in perception and understanding. The path of Brahma-charya, then, cannot be chosen just because it is something very glamorous or just to be different from other people.

Throughout life we make decisions, and the decisions we make focus our lives in the direction in which we want to go. It starts already with young people deciding whether to quit school at fourteen or sixteen, or to go on to university; whether to earn just a B.A. or to take a Ph.D. When a clear decision is made and all energies are focused in that direction, one will be a success in one's chosen career. If the focus is on Self-knowledge and Liberation, on the powers and mysteries of the mind, then events will shift accordingly.

The decisions about sex, love, and marriage need to be made with at least as much care as when one buys a car or a house. How dependable is the car mechanically? How comfortable and how affordable is the house? What is my motivation for marriage? In general, what kind of a person do I want to be—physically, mentally, spiritually? What is the purpose of my life? What should my life be, so that it will be worthwhile living? All these questions have to lead to a discussion with oneself. It is important to remember that celibacy is not just practiced by single people, aspiring yogis, monks and nuns, but by quite a number of other people who shift their focus for longer or shorter periods of time to different goals. It may not be public knowledge that players of professional sports are kept on strict celibacy for a couple of weeks before the season begins to be able to concentrate all their physical energy on the game.

While there may be those within a marriage relationship who would like to seek spiritual attainment, divided interests prevent the single-pointedness that is necessary for success. For such people, a realistic view of the pursuit of Yoga would be to gain a balance of mental and emotional health, to lay a solid foundation for the time when they can devote themselves entirely to the spiritual life. Until that time, celibacy is looked upon as unnecessary or even unhealthy.

B.K.S. Iyengar, in *Light on Yoga,* gives a detailed description of the asanas which will cure impotence and sterility, and those which can be practiced for Brahmacharya.[1] The preserving of sexual energy creates a powerful and radiant personality, making the brahmachari even more desirable to the opposite sex. The increased physical and mental powers resulting from Brahmacharya have to be used wisely. Wendy Doniger O'Flaherty, in her various writings, tells many delightful stories of Parvati and Shiva when he or she was the ascetic or when he or she was the erotic, illustrating the potential use of accumulated power.

According to the *Hatha-Yoga-Pradipika,* "Only a Yogin leading the life of a Brahmacharin and observing a moderate and nutritious diet, obtains perfection in the manipulation of Kundalini within forty-five days."[2] And, "Consider him not to be a Brahmacharin, but an utter failure in Yoga, and subject to old age, death and all sorts of infirmities as long as he has not controlled his seminal essence, and attained the state of samadhi. Such a man is said to be worldly."[3] In the *Bhagavad Gita,* VI:14: "Serene-minded, fearless, firm in the vow of a Brahmachari, having controlled the mind, thinking of Me and balanced in mind, let him sit, having Me as his supreme goal." And in VIII:11: "That which is declared imperishable by those who know the Vedas, that which the self-controlled (ascetics or Sanyasins) and passion-free enter, that desiring which celibacy is practised—that goal I will declare to thee in brief." And again in XVII:14: "Worship of the gods, the twice-born, the teachers and the wise, purity, straightforwardness, celibacy and non-injury are called the austerities of the body."

It might be remembered that Jesus said that in heaven there are no marriages. He also said, "Follow me" and "Be ye perfect as your Father in heaven is perfect." That perfection is not very well understood, and there is much argument about it. Can such perfection be obtained in one lifetime? And does it not require single-pointed focus of attention? Jesus said, too, that a man who followed a woman with lustful eyes had already committed a sin. And the Book of Revelations says, "You have foregone your first love . . . for God."

We may or may not accept scriptural texts of any kind as indeed being the word of God, and take the attitude that, regardless of the divine inspiration that may have been the true author, those written words have passed through the mind of an individual and been tainted by it. And yet, the essential message in all religions has been, Be good, do good, be compassionate, be honest, do not injure others.

But human inconsistency, frailty, need for change, or development in different directions, have contributed to seeking answers to the problems that arise from this interplay of forces. We can achieve much through the practice of Yoga. Acquiring a good state of health on the physical and mental-emotional level, we may come closer to the given potential. Some might even be able to reawaken the forces of self-healing; and there will also be some who recognize the body as a spiritual tool and allow their own heart to become a center of awe and wonder at this incredible cosmic force for which human beings have so many different names, and for which they create so many astounding forms.

Sexual activity as essential to physical health has been a controversy among many people. Dr. R. S. Mishra, a Sanskrit scholar who is trained in medicine and psychiatry, says, "Brahmacharya, continence, is a protection of hormonal power by controlling sex impetus. That means not only abstinence from sexual intercourse, but also abstinence from sexual thinking and impulses. Male and female seeds are the highest productive energy. They should be used only for productive purposes."[4] And "A hungry man thinks pictorially, and dreams about eating. Likewise a man in sexual desire thinks in pictures, and dreams about sex."[5] Once more we become aware that there is much cause for wrong identification and that wrong identification leads one astray. Identifying with a feeling like love, hatred, or anger, or with the sexual drive, means that the Light is no longer present. The need to transcend personality aspects and to identify with the Light is now obvious. "I am not the body, I am not the mind, I am eternal Light."[6]

Dr. Mishra gives clear direction by saying, "A person having lust and desire understands every person of the opposite sex as an object of sex and, due to this relationship, hankering and its consequences come upon him. A student of Self-realization understands every object, every member, as a manifestation of the Supreme, and due to change of relationship, happiness and its consequences come to him. Here objects are not destroyed; only the relationships are changed."[7] And also, "Having reached a higher state, a yogin begins to receive cosmic suggestions and his individual suggestions gradually stop."[8]

Self-observation and self-analysis in Yoga are not limited to technical use as in Western psychology. They are not possible without really involving the Self; however, in the beginning involvement will be mainly with the personality aspects. To investigate and analyze anything and everything is very helpful, but it cannot end there. In the field of Yoga one has to look over all the territory, all the worlds in which one lives. The objective must not be criticism, or to become clever to avoid criticism, but to indeed know oneself. Psychoanalysis as practiced today is not sufficient. It has to reach the level of Self-recognition.

Dr. Mishra warns that psychoanalysis or self-analysis should not be confined to any particular doctrine. He feels that religions and their sects are already overwhelmed with too many doctrines and too many dogmas.

Gandhi's views on marriage and Brahmacharya are well-known. He has put out ten rules, which are here included.

1. Boys and girls should be brought up simply and naturally in the full belief that they are and can remain innocent.

2. All should abstain from heating and stimulating foods.

3. Husband and wife should occupy separate rooms and avoid privacy.

4. Both body and mind should be constantly and healthily occupied.

5. Early to bed and early to rise should be strictly observed.

6. All unclean literature should be avoided.

7. Theatres, cinemas, etc., which tend to stimulate passion should be shunned.

8. Nocturnal dreams need not cause any anxiety. A cold bath every time for a fairly strong person is the finest preventive in such cases.

9. Above all, one must not consider continence even as between husband and wife to be so difficult as to be practically impossible.

10. A heart-felt prayer every day for purity makes one progressively pure.[9]

Dependence and interdependence become more obvious when the desire for Cosmic Consciousness has reached a point where it has diminished all other desires. Milarepa, the great Tibetan yogi, is reported as having achieved this incredible feat in one lifetime; and yet there is reference to the fact that the karmic conditions were right. It has been made clear by all the writers of the various texts that it takes many lifetimes even to acquire such a desire. It is necessary in each lifetime to do the utmost to be at some time in such a state of blessing that the last phase can be completed.

1.   The following asanas are cited in *Light on Yoga* for controlling the sex drive: Pascimottanasana (166-170); Parivrtta Pascimottanasana (170-173); Mulabandhasana (344-346); Kandasana (348-352); Supta Trivikramasana (356-357); Eka Pada Rajakapotasana cycle (389-395); Rajakapotasana (398).

2.   *Hatha-Yoga-Pradipika,* 71.

3.   Ibid., 106.

4.   Mishra, *Textbook of Yoga Psychology,* 199.

5.   Ibid., 166.

6.   Sivananda Radha, *Divine Light Invocation.*

7.   Mishra, *Textbook of Yoga Psychology,* 320.

8.   Ibid., 228.

9.   Gandhi, *The Law of Continence,* 102-103.

ASANAS: The Hidden Language

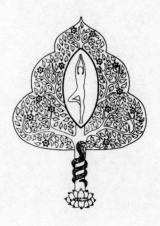

conclusion

ASANAS: The Hidden Language

CONCERN FOR THE HUMAN condition and recognition of the complexity of human life, not only in the East but also for the Westerner, have led me to take this step—to attempt to build a bridge between Western psychology and Yoga Psychology, using the symbolism of Hatha Yoga asanas.

To blend East and West, we can take what is valuable in the West and put it together with yogic philosophy and methods. Western psychology, particularly Transpersonal Psychology, is a stepping-stone to the analysis that is done by the Easterner through the application of Yoga Psychology.

We can use Western methods such as free thought association, and investigate ourselves by observing others, then figuring out where the same thing exists in us. But this is only a small beginning. Investigating these things and the way your mind works leads to knowing yourself better, but this is not what is called "sadhana" in the East.[1] Even Yoga Psychology is not sadhana; it is a preparation. True sadhana is the third step. It is your spiritual practice, reflection, and, to some extent, your dreams, if you use them to understand the unconscious and if you see the dreams of sleep as not much different from those of the day. You may learn that it is possible to alter the content of your sleep-dreams as much as you can alter your daydreams or your dreams of life.

Asana practice is part of sadhana and can be done at the same time that you do the necessary psychological work on yourself. By using Western methods and Yoga Psychology, you will recognize what you have to do, and understand why your sadhana is the step that follows. Sadhana is meant to take you to the Divine. The psychological work is the means to do your sadhana more peacefully, so it will be more effective and so you can enter a different state of mind at will. The object of sadhana is to live in the Divine Consciousness and to manifest it in life; but this is possible only if, at the same time, daily reflection is done with an openness to new insights. Should you make the choice to tap those inner resources for the spiritual significance of the asanas, the methods given in this book can be pondered and enlarged, and used to discover greater personal meaning.

If one could do sadhana like Milarepa,[2] who did nothing else in life, insights would come—but it would still take years. Even in his situation it took many years. In each lifetime one gains a little, but one loses also. That is a very slow process. The Easterner usually thinks in terms of hundreds of lifetimes to reach Liberation, but Milarepa thought differently; he told people they could achieve Higher Consciousness in one lifetime if they could break their attachments. By using the methods of Transpersonal Psychology and Yoga Psychology, we zero in on the problems and try to deal with them, and that can save many lifetimes.

Traditional Western psychology can be said to be a first step in the process of awareness. However, shifting the emphasis from one personality aspect to another cannot be seen as a solution. Whereas Western psychology aims at adaptation to the world—social, economic, and domestic survival—Yoga Psychology deals with developing potential and the discovery and unfolding of the Divine within. Transpersonal Psychology, with its goal of embracing the human being as a physical body and as a mental-emotional entity, and with its use of some methods for transcending personality aspects, seems to be the most accessible bridge for the Westerner to the psychology and philosophy of the East.

Some of the Buddhist texts tell us that the four powers meant to be used by a disciple to achieve purification are: sincere repentance; determination not to do the same thing again; the understanding of good deeds and compensation for wrong actions; and contemplating the void of the nature of being. Transpersonal Psychology, in combination with Yoga Psychology, will bring these things to the individual's attention and then the decision can be made to counteract them with various spiritual practices, such as Hatha Yoga.

The old tradition of Yoga is that one has to do one's sadhana to achieve a new consciousness, one that will surpass the power of reasoning and the power of the intellect, so that both can be controlled every step of the way. Through the self-examination that was stressed by my Guru and the other Gurus that I have met, one can see and experience what needs to be corrected. Yoga Psychology puts one through a process that shows exactly what needs to be done; the direct experience has no substitute. That is the purpose of the whole process of Kundalini Yoga (which includes Hatha Yoga)—to lay the foundation through personal experience. Sadhana in conjunction with Yoga Psychology is cooperation with the course of evolution.

If, prior to working out all psychological problems, spiritual practice is difficult, you should persist regardless, either by sheer will power or by making the choice to remove the obstacles. Your mind then becomes very fertile ground. You can relate that to the plough posture: you plough through your own life, through your own being, through your many personality aspects and realize what they are. By so doing you have prepared the ground for an effective or successful sadhana.

The emphasis on the psychological aspects will make you acquainted with them. You then have a choice of letting them rule you or not. You cannot entirely eliminate them. You will always have the aspect of being a father, husband, mother or wife, co-worker, etc.; but unless you look at yourself in these roles, you do not know what a large part they play in hostile or harmonious interaction with others. Each personality aspect is loaded with opinions, convictions, and beliefs that can cause many difficulties.

We have an advantage in having some understanding of

Western psychology, particularly Transpersonal Psychology. By using the methods of guided imagery and guided association, we can lead our thinking into deeper levels. When you look into a garden pool, for instance, you may comment on the lovely lilies or fish, but you do not usually think further. But if I ask you to think in depth about the fish posture, you can consider that a person can be in the water—but for how long? You can't live in the water, whereas the fish can. The fish can't come out of the water; in order for it to live out of the water it has to follow a line of evolution that you as a human being have left behind. The memory of that time in your evolution now remains only in the first four or five months of being an embryo in the uterine environment (you still have webbed feet and hands at this stage). The stories of water babies and mermaids are all a reminder from mythology of how the past has evolved into the present.

Mythology is a mirroring of our past and, as we move on, the past recedes more and more into the background. These images are still valid, but need to be investigated to discover their meaning now. For example, in the case of the mermaid, does she represent areas where I am neither fish nor human? Or does she mean that I can adapt to either environment? What is my relationship to the lotus and the lily and to the fish? In thinking about water, you can see that you live in an element of life that is like a big ocean; there are many creatures, some of which are friendly and some hostile. By using the outlines given in this book for the asanas, you are taken through a process to a point at which you realize that you are not an island; you live in a world in which there are many forms of life. You become more accepting of those you live amongst. In the urban environment, in a world in which you are one person among many, having one tiny place and no right to demand more, you do not usually think of your relationship to your surroundings. All of the asanas, except for the structural ones, have names from the different animal and vegetable kingdoms because that is the world in which human beings find themselves. Through working with these symbols we can understand that many of their characteristics are also ours.

In ancient times people also used symbols from the world around them. Lecterns in old churches have been decorated with images of the ox, the lion, the eagle, and the angel to symbolize the four evangelists. Mark was represented as a lion with a halo around him, standing on a book. We can assume from this symbolism that Mark was a forceful person who had control over people, and that he was probably a powerful orator when he talked about Jesus' teachings. His power is symbolized by the roar of the lion. He is shown as being strong, rather than ferocious, by the halo and by the fact that he is standing on the Book of Knowledge. John is symbolized by the eagle; he has sharp, penetrating understanding—an eagle can see from very far away. Matthew is shown as an angel with a halo and the Book of Life. The halo means a much higher state of consciousness, which he attained by the sharpness of his intellect. Most Christians do not know that the evangelists were ever represented in this way. The modern church has little resemblance to the older one, in which symbolism was used and understood. The symbol of Jesus as a lamb, willing to be sacrificed, however, is a familiar one; there is nothing extraordinary about it. But we pay little attention to symbolism, so when we come in contact with different symbols and different metaphors, we look on them as something strange.

When we become aware of symbolism we may realize that, although meanings can be slightly different in different cultures, they retain their strong influences. For example, the old churches were built in the shape of a cross representing sacrifice; but it can also mean being on the crossroads of life. One moves up to the crossroads, to the fourth chakra of the Kundalini system, and then decides if one is satisfied with just being a nice person, or if one wants to go all the way.

Symbolism explains something that is difficult to put into

ASANAS: The Hidden Language

words. This is particularly true of the Teachings, since they have come from a time when writing and reading were available to only a very few. Human beings live much more by symbol and metaphor than they realize. (There is a billion dollar industry in advertizing built on the use of symbols.) They are marvelous tools for understanding the functioning of the mind and the responses from powerful emotions, as you will have seen in working with the symbols of the asanas.

Foreign tissue in the human body is fought fiercely as an invading organism; but so also are fought invading thoughts, invading philosophical systems. Although most people are still very mechanical in their thinking and reactions, there are always a few who are truly interested in the mysteries of life and of the mind. These courageous few are willing to investigate the ancient Teachings to find out how they can apply in their own lives today. The old texts were meant to guide people through their lives, to help them know and understand better how to live, how to improve the capacity of the senses and the mind.

It is difficult to investigate the mind because the mind itself is its own tool. It is also difficult to investigate language because the spoken word is the tool. There is more speculation than knowledge concerning language, as there is little recorded history. It is said that the Vedas were written about 3000 B.C., when the rishis recognized that the power of the human mind was declining and it would therefore be necessary to record those ancient hymns in order to preserve them. Up to that time people's memories were so good that the Teachings were passed on orally. Whether this was the beginning of written language is hard to say, but from my own practices and experiences, I know that language is related to consciousness, and for consciousness to evolve it was necessary for language to evolve. Poetry has a special place in the language of any culture. It avoids reducing language to a use that is only practical, for communication or conversation, socializing, intellectualizing, theorizing. There is a different spirit in every word. Language can deal with the ordinary, but it can also deal with that higher expression that goes on in the mind, as well as the inner sacred life expressed by the phrase, "the still, small voice within."

Traditional ways have served their purpose in the past. Those who are traditionalists will resist change and be critical of any new approach, but ways of life do evolve. The meanings of words change within a culture, as they do also from one culture to another. While the scholar is concerned about the original meaning of a word, that word may no longer mean the same thing in general usage; for instance, the word *awful* used to mean "inspiring awe"; now it is commonly used as the equivalent to "very bad" or "terrible."

When scholars told me that I did not pronounce the Mantra correctly, I said, "It works." And I told them the story of my Guru, Swami Sivananda, asking the people around him, who came from different parts of India, to say his name. He pointed out that he always knew that they meant him regardless of how they pronounced it. The image that is created in the mind is the deciding factor.

It is ridiculous to insist that words have to maintain certain meanings regardless of the century and culture in which they are used. It would render old philosophical ideas useless if they could not be made meaningful today. We must begin in the place where we are because it is from there that we can make another step. Although we cannot accept on faith the vision of the seers or rishis of ancient times that the Divine Word is Brahman,[3] the understanding of that insight has to be the goal. To know the vocabulary of one's own conscious mind as well as the unconscious, and to see how we use language to manipulate ourselves and others, will bring about increased comprehension of the power of speech.

A wonderful example from the Eastern Teachings of changes in words used to express a meaning is the symbol of the swan, which in the West was substituted for the Indian goose because in European countries to call someone a goose is rather degrading. The chattering of the goose is often applied

ASANAS: The Hidden Language

to people, especially women, who chatter in the marketplace as they sell their wares. The word *goose* was replaced because the swan is a very majestic and aesthetic concept for the Western mind.

From the accumulation of life experience throughout the ages, mythology reveals truth in a very particular language —one could almost say a forgotten language. We know little about meanings, symbols, and metaphors, because we float on the surface of life like a leaf on the surface of the waves, too involved in worldly affairs to investigate deeply. The ancients obviously lived by symbol and metaphor, and we could profit today by rediscovering that symbol and metaphor in the Teachings of the East.

If any Teachings are to be kept alive in another culture, the different social setting in which they originated must be taken into consideration. Many Indian Gurus have appeared in the West, but what is tolerated in their country may be looked at with suspicion in this country and be open to sharp criticism. Those cultural differences will always be present, but if we are concerned mainly with keeping the Teachings alive, we must realize that anything that is brought from another country is open to adaptation and reinterpretation in a new culture. There will be some loss, but there will also be some gain. Not all Yogic Teachings from the past are adaptable to the Western culture, perhaps not even to modern India.

The impact today of the influence of the Eastern philosophies here in the West has stirred up great concern among orthodox institutions. But it is forgotten that Western missionaries have gone to the East and created the same kind of confusion, difficulties, and disruption to families. The resulting Christianity is not the same as it is here, but neither is Western Christianity the same as it was a thousand years ago. And if Westerners were to go to the Holy Land they would find that the descendents of the ancient Gnostics resemble American Christians very little.

In an interview the Dalai Lama said that there is Chinese Buddhism, Japanese Buddhism, Tibetan Buddhism, and there will be American, or French, or Canadian Buddhism, because whatever a disciple gets from a Guru becomes incorporated in the disciple's makeup, understanding, and personality. Each Guru will attract those who are at the level to understand the language by which the two will communicate. But, as with anything, there is always a higher level. In my previous book, *Kundalini: Yoga for the West,* it was emphasized that laying of the foundation (character building) is only the first step. Meditation, Mantra chanting, Hatha Yoga will improve character and bring quality into life. Theory alone leads just to intellectualization, which does not improve anybody's life. Pandits or scholars can make little contribution to the pursuit of the path of Yoga, except intellectually or in theory, which is perhaps only for the pleasure of a handful of people who enjoy the elegance of the pure traditional presentation

In the Eastern tradition, the great yogis of the past have often been transformed in the minds of people into beings more extraordinary than they in fact were. This is similar to what we read of the lives of saints in the West. There is barely ever any mention of character traits that made life difficult in monasteries, or of the undercurrents in monasteries of both the East and West. The theory presented regarding the perfection of these beings has little meaning to us. The need to preserve this image of perfection is only for the few who want to keep this on an intellectual level, leather-bound on their bookshelves, well removed from the nitty-gritty of daily life.

On the other hand, there is a tendency in the West to elevate people to superhuman status and then to strip them down by exposing their psychological idiosyncfacies. Winston Churchill was reduced to a normal human being by having his weaknesses exposed, and now the same thing is being done to Freud.

Perhaps being clear and direct, not glorifying or reducing

ASANAS: The Hidden Language

anyone, but seeing these lives as something that we can learn from, would serve our purposes better. In old Europe, the saints' lives first served as an example; later, doctrines developed around their lives and personalities. But the description of the struggle and lives of saintly individuals has much more to offer to those who want to find meaning and purpose in life. The personal lives of the saints, East or West, were unorthodox, and their personality aspects, when seen as a whole, often did not fit into the society in which they found themselves. It takes a great deal of courage to be different, because people feel uneasy about such individuals and take every opportunity to attack them.

The Gurus I have met agreed with the old rishis who emphasized an approach aimed at the practical achievement of a spiritual goal, a vision of the Divine as a result of practical application of the Teachings, rather than intellectual speculation.

An important question that comes up over and over is whether students of Yoga should learn Sanskrit. A natural inclination or desire should be encouraged when it is not limited to an intellectual interest. What counts is the motivation and the understanding gained. Christians have never been encouraged to learn Aramaic or ancient Hebrew or Greek to understand the origin of their religion. Although there is an advantage in reading a text in its original language, it would be very difficult to put oneself back into that era to know, for example, what the Jews were like at the time of Christ, how they thought about words and incidents. The late Dr. Lamsa, whose native language was Aramaic and who wrote *Light on the Gospels,* was amazed at what modern Christians had done with the Teachings, and the way events that are still seen as very common affairs in the Holy Land had been turned into miracles. Something similar is happening now with the Indian and Tibetan Teachings, and I appreciate the Dalai Lama's understanding that the Western mind will have a different grasp of them.

ASANAS: The Hidden Language

As Westerners we have to start within our own culture and go as far as we can with Western psychology, using some of the yogic approach. The psychological work of recognizing personality aspects, learning self-acceptance, and stripping away illusions, opens the door for understanding and applying Yoga Psychology. Sadhana will then come easily. The aim has now gone beyond becoming a better person in order to get along with family or co-workers, to make life smooth. The goal now is to become what Swami Sivananda called an all-round developed, harmonious human being, to bring you closer to the realization of the divinity within yourself—to achieve the state of God- or Self-realization.

It is easy to state that all is unreal and that Consciousness alone is real; but to understand this, if it does not happen in a sudden flash, is possible only through what can be called a clearing process. If the Teachings elevate, inspire, or benefit you, and if you are prepared to do the necessary work, that is all that is needed to start. It is my hope that this new approach to the asanas of Hatha Yoga will help you to develop the potential that is waiting within you to be tapped.

1. Serving the Divine through spiritual practice.

2. See *Halasana: Plough,* page 89, reference note 8.

3. "The world of sound is described in Sanskrit as the manifestation of Brahman, the Divine or Absolute Being." Tyberg, *Language of the Gods,* 17.

bibliography

Adamson, Joy. *Born Free: A Lioness of Two Worlds.* London: Collins & Harvil Press, 1960.

————. *Living Free: The Story of Elsa and Her Cubs.* London: Collins & Harvil Press, 1961.

Ancient Egypt: Discovering Its Splendors. Washington D.C.: National Geographic Society, 1978.

"The Anugita." In *Sacred Books of the East.* Vol. 8. 1882. Reprint. Delhi: Motilal Banarsidass, 1975.

Ashwell, Reg. *Coast Salish.* Saanichton, B.C.: Hancock House, 1978.

Avalon, Arthur. *Ananda Lahari. (Wave of Bliss).* 4th ed. Madras: Ganesh & Co., 1953.

Bachofen, J. J. *Myth, Religion, & Mother Right.* Bollingen Series. Translated by Ralph Manheim. Princeton: Princeton University Press, 1967.

Bakan, David. "Belief and the management of chronic pain." *Journal of Humanistic Psychology,* 20 (Fall 1980) no. 4:37-44.

Bayley, Harold. *The Lost Language of Symbolism.* 1912. Reprint. New Jersey: Rowman & Littlefield, 1974.

Bernard, Theos. *Heaven Lies Within Us.* London: Rider & Co., 1952.

Beyer, Stephan. *The Cult of Tara.* Berkeley: University of California Press, 1973.

The Bhagavad Gita. Translated by Swami Sivananda. 9th ed. Rishikesh, India: Divine Life Society, 1982.

The Bhagavadgita With the Sanatsujatiya and the Anugita. Vol. 8 of *Sacred Books of the East.* Translated by K. T. Telang. 1882. Reprint. Delhi: Motilal Banarsidass, 1975.

The Bhagavata Purana. Vol. 10 of *Ancient Indian Tradition and Mythology.* Edited by J. L. Shastri. Delhi: Motilal Banarsidass, 1978.

Bhattacharyya, D. C. *Tantric Buddhist Iconographic Sources.* New Delhi: Munshiram Manoharlal, 1974.

Bonner, J. T. *Evolution of Culture in Animals*. Princeton: Princeton University Press, 1981.

Brenneman Jr., Walter L. *Spirals: A Study in Symbol, Myth & Ritual*. Washington, D.C.: University Press of America Inc., 1979.

Brown, Gabrielle. *The New Celibacy*. New York: Ballantine Books, 1980.

Brown, Joseph Epes. "Sun dance: sacrifice, renewal, identity." *Parabola,* 3(2): 12-15, May 1978.

Budge, E. A. Wallis. *Amulets & Talismans*. Reprint. New York: University Books, 1968.

————. *The Egyptian Heaven and Hell*. LaSalle, Ill.: Open Court Publishing Co., 1905.

————. *The Egyptian Book of the Dead*. 1895. Reprint. New York: Dover Publications, 1967.

————. *Gods of the Egyptians*. 2 vols. 1904. Reprint. New York: Dover Publications, 1969.

Burland, Cottie and Werner Forman. *Gods and Fate in Ancient Mexico*. Orbis Publ. Ltd., 1975.

Campbell, Joseph. *The Masks of God: Creative Mythology*. New York: Viking Press, 1968.

————. *The Masks of God: Occidental Mythology*. New York: Viking Press, 1964.

————. *The Masks of God: Oriental Mythology*. New York: Viking Press, 1962.

————. *The Masks of God: Primitive Mythology*. New York: Viking Press, 1959.

————. *The Mythic Image*. Bollingen Series C. Princeton: Princeton University Press, 1974.

Cavendish, Richard. *Visions of Heaven and Hell*. New York: Harmony Books, 1977.

Churchward, Albert. *The Signs and Symbols of Primordial Man*. 2d ed. London: George Allen & Co., 1913.

Cirlot, J. E. *A Dictionary of Symbols*. New York: Philosophical Library, 1962.

Classical Hindu Mythology. Edited and translated by Cornelia Dimmitt and J. A. D. van Buitenen. Philadelphia: Temple University Press, 1978.

Coomaraswamy, Ananda K. & Sister Nivedita. *Myths of the Hindus and Buddhists*. 1913. Reprint. New York: Dover Publications, 1967.

Coomaraswamy. I: Selected Papers, Traditional Art and Symbolism. Edited by Roger Lipsey. Bollingen Series 89. Princeton: Princeton University Press, 1977.

Cooper, J. C. *Illustrated Encyclopaedia of Traditional Symbols*. London: Thames and Hudson, 1978.

The Crucible of Christianity. Edited by Arnold Toynbee. London: Thames and Hudson, 1969.

D'Alviella, Goblet. *The Migration of Symbols*. 1892. Reprint. Wellingborough: The Aquarian Press, 1979.

DeVries, Ad. *Dictionary of Symbols and Imagery*. Amsterdam: North Holland Publishers, 1974.

Dowson, John. *A Classical Dictionary of Hindu Mythology*. 12th ed. London: Routledge & Kegan Paul, 1972.

Dutt, S. *Buddhist Monks and Monasteries of India*. New York: Fernhill House, 1962.

Edwards, I. E. S. *Tutankhamun: His Tomb and Its Treasures*. New York: Metropolitan Museum of Art & Alfred A. Knopf, 1977.

Eliade, Mircea. *Cosmos and History: The Myth of the Eternal Return*. 1954. Reprint. New York: Harper & Brothers, 1959.

————. *Myths, Dreams and Mysteries*. Translated by Philip Maaret. New York: Harper & Row, 1960.

Eliot, Alexander. *Myths*. New York: McGraw-Hill Book Co., 1976.

Encyclopedia of World Mythology. London: Octopus Books, 1975.

Evans-Wentz, W. Y. *Cuchama and Sacred Mountains*. Chicago: Swallow Press, 1981.

————. *Tibet's Great Yogi Milarepa*. 1928. Reprint. London: Oxford University Press, 1969.

————. *The Tibetan Book of the Dead*. 3d ed. London: Oxford University Press, 1957.

Feuerstein, Georg. *Textbook of Yoga*. London: Rider and Co., 1975.

Firth, Violet. [Dion Fortune, pseud.] *The Problem of Purity*. New York: Samuel Weiser, n.d.

————. *The Esoteric Philosophy of Love and Marriage*. London: Aquarian Press, 1957.

Fisher, Helen E. *The Sex Contract: The Evolution of Human Behavior.* New York: William Morrow & Co., 1982.

Frazer, James G. *Folklore in the Old Testament.* New York: Hart Publishing Co., 1975.

————. *The Golden Bough.* Abridged ed. London: Macmillan & Co., 1963.

Freible, Charles. "Teilhard, sexual love, and celibacy." *Review for Religions,* 26(1967): 282-294.

Freund, Philip. *Myths of Creation.* 1964. Reprint. New York: Transatlantic Arts, Inc., 1975.

Gandhi, M. K. *An Autobiography: The Story of My Experiments With Truth.* Boston: Beacon Press, 1968.

————. *The Law of Continence: Brahmacharya.* Edited by Anand T. Hingorani. Bombay: Bharatiya Vidya Bhavan, 1964.

Gaskell, G. A. *Dictionary of All Scriptures and Myths.* New York: Julian Press, 1960.

The Gheranda Samhita. Translated by Sris Chandra Vasu. Adyar: Theosophical Publishing House, 1933.

Gibran, Kahlil. *The Prophet.* 1923. Reprint. New York: Alfred A. Knopf, 1958.

Gordon, Antoinette K. *The Iconography of Tibetan Lamaism.* rev. ed. Rutland, Vt.: Charles E. Tuttle Co., 1959.

Govinda, Lama Anagarika. *The Way of the White Clouds.* 1966. Reprint. Boston: Shambhala Publications, 1972.

Graves, Robert. *The White Goddess.* Amended and enlarged. New York: Vintage Books, 1959.

Green, Elmer and Alyce M. "On the meaning of transpersonal: some metaphysical perspectives." *Journal of Transpersonal Psychology,* 3(1971) no. 1: 37.

————. *Beyond Biofeedback.* New York: Dell Publishing Co., 1977.

Grelot, Pierre. *Man and Wife in Scripture.* New York: Herder and Herder, 1964.

Gubernatis, Angelo de. *Zoological Mythology.* 2 vols. New York: Arno Press, 1978.

Guenther, H. V. and L. S. Kawamura. *Mind in Buddhist Psychology.* Emeryville, Calif.: Dharma Publishing, 1975.

Gustafson, Janie. *Celibate Passion.* San Francisco: Harper & Row, 1978.

Haich, Elisabeth. *Sexual Energy and Yoga.* New York: ASI Publishers, 1972.

Hammond, N. G. L. and H. H. Scullard. *The Oxford Classical Dictionary.* 2d ed. London: Oxford University Press, 1970.

The Hathayogapradipika. Translated by Srinivasa Iyangar. 3d ed. Ayar, India: Theosophical Publishing House, 1949.

Herrigel, Eugen. *Zen in the Art of Archery.* New York: Vintage Books, 1971.

Hindu Myths. With an introduction by Wendy Doniger O'Flaherty. New York: Penguin Books, 1975.

Hutchinson, R. W. *Prehistoric Crete.* Baltimore, Md.: Penguin Books, 1962.

The I Ching. 3d ed. Translated by Richard Wilhelm. Princeton: Princeton University Press, 1967.

The Illiad of Homer. Translated by Richmond Lattimore. 1951. Reprint. Chicago: University of Chicago Press, 1976.

The Indian Mind: Essentials of Indian Philosophy and Culture. Edited by Charles A. Moore. Honolulu: University Press of Hawaii, 1977.

Iyengar, B. K. S. *Light on Pranayama.* New York: The Crossroad Publishing Co., 1981.

———. *Light on Yoga.* rev. ed. New York: Schocken Books, 1977.

———. *Sparks of Divinity.* Paris: Institut de Yoga B. K. S. Iyengar, 1976.

———. *Iyengar: His Life and Work.* Porthill, Idaho: Timeless Books, 1987.

Johnson, Robert A. *She: Understanding Feminine Psychology.* New York: Harper & Row, 1977.

Jordan-Smith, Paul. "The breath of Brahma." *Parabola,* 2(3): 53, 1977.

Khan, Mohammad I. *Sarasvati in Sanscrit Literature.* Ghasiabad, India: Crescent Publishing House, 1978.

Kiesling, Christopher. "Celibacy, friendship and prayer." *Review for Religions,* 30 (1971): 595-617.

Kuvalayananda, Swami. *Asanas.* 1933. Reprint. Lonavala, India: Kaivalyadhama, 1977.

———. *Yoga Therapy.* 1963. Reprint. New Delhi: Central Health Education Bureau, Ministry of Health, 1971.

Kyselka, Will and Ray Lanterman. *North Star to Southern Cross.* 1976. Reprint. Honolulu: University Press of Hawaii, 1980.

Lamy, Lucie. *Egyptian Mysteries.* Crossroad Publishing Co., 1981.

Larousse World Mythology. Edited by Pierre Grimal. London: Paul Hamlyn, 1971.

Lauf, Detlef Ingo. *Secret Doctrines of the Tibetan Books of the Dead.* Boulder: Shambhala Publishers, 1977.

Lea, Henry C. *The History of Sacerdotal Celibacy in the Christian Church.* New York: Russell & Russell, 1957.

Lehane, Brendan. *The Power of Plants.* Maidenhead, England: McGraw-Hill Book Co., 1977.

The Li Ki. Sacred Books of China. Vol. 27 of *Sacred Books of the East.* Translated by James Legge. 1885. Reprint. Delhi: Motilal Banarsidass, 1976.

Life and Its Marvels. Englewood Cliffs, N. J.: International Graphic Society, 1960.

Life-Nature Library: The Birds. By Roger T. Peterson. New York: Time-Life Books, 1963.

Life-Nature Library: The Desert. By A. Starker Leopold. New York: Time-Life Books, 1961.

Life-Nature Library: The Fishes. By F. D. Ommanney. New York: Time-Life Books, 1963.

Life-Nature Library: The Insects. By Peter Farb. New York: Time-Life Books, 1962.

Life-Nature Library: The Reptiles. By Archie Carr. New York: Time-Life Books, 1963.

The Lion's Roar of Queen Srimala. Translated by Alex and Hideko Wayman. New York: Columbia University Press, 1974.

Maculloch, John A. *The Mythology of All Races.* Vol. 2. Cooper Square Publishers, 1922.

Maslow, Abraham. "A philosophy of psychology." Reprinted from *Personal Problems and Psychological Frontiers.* Edited by J. Fairchild. Sheridan House Press, 1957.

McBride, Chris. *The White Lions of Timbavati.* New York: Paddington Press, 1977.

"The meaning of death." In *Coomaraswamy. II: Selected Papers. Metaphysics.* Edited by Roger Lipsey. Princeton: Princeton University Press, 1977.

Michanowsky, George. *The Once and Future Star.* Reprint. New York: Barnes & Noble, 1977.

Mishra, Rammurti S. *The Textbook of Yoga Psychology.* New York: Julian Press, 1963.

The Mountain Spirit. Edited by Michael C. Tobias and H. Drasdo. Woodstock, N.Y.: Overlook Press, 1979.

"The Mundaka Upanishad." In *The Thirteen Principal Upanishads.* 2d ed. rev. Translated by Robert E. Hume. London: Oxford University Press, 1931.

Narada Maha Thera. *A Manual of Abhidhamma.* 4th ed. Sri Lanka: Publication Society, 1980.

Neumann, Erich. *The Great Mother.* 2d ed. Bollingen Series 47. Princeton: Princeton University Press, 1963.

"Now that I come to die." Translated by Herbert V. Guenther. *Crystal Mirror,* 5: 331-343, 1977.

The Ocean of Story. Translated by C. H. Tawney, edited by N. M. Penzer. 10 vols. 2d rev. ed. Delhi: Motilal Banarsidass, 1924.

Ochs, Carol. *Behind the Sex of God.* Boston: Beacon Press, 1977.

The Odyssey of Homer. Translated by Richmond Lattimore. 1965. Reprint. Harper & Row, 1977.

O'Flaherty, Wendy D. *Asceticism & Eroticism in the Mythology of Siva.* London: Oxford University Press, 1973.

———. *The Origins of Evil in Hindu Mythology.* Berkeley: University of California Press, 1976.

———. *Women, Androgynes, and Other Mythical Beasts.* Chicago: University of Chicago Press, 1980.

Packard, Vance. *The Sexual Wilderness.* New York: David McKay Co., 1968.

Parrinder, Geoffrey. *Sex in the World's Religions.* Don Mills, Ont.: General Publishing Co. Ltd., 1980.

Peck, William H. *Egyptian Drawings.* New York: E. P. Dutton, 1978.

Pelletier, K. R. *Mind as Healer, Mind as Slayer.* New York: Delta Books, 1977.

The Penguin Book of World Folk Tales. Edited by Milton Rugoff. 1949. Reprint. New York: Penguin Books, 1977.

Phelan, Nancy and Michael Volin. *Sex and Yoga.* New York: Harper & Row, 1968.

Platt, Rutherford. *A Pocket Guide to Trees.* New York: Washington Square Press, 1960.

Purce, Jill. *The Mystic Spiral: Journey of the Soul.* New York: Avon Books, 1974.

The Questions of King Milinda. Vols. 35 & 36 of *Sacred Books of the East.* Translated by T. W. Rhys Davids. 1894. Reprint. Delhi: Motilal Banarsidass, 1975.

Radhakrishnan. *The Hindu View of Life.* New York: Macmillan Co., 1969.

Raja, C. Kunhan. "Asya Vamasya Hymn" (The Riddle of the Universe). *Rigveda,* 1-164. Madras: Ganesh & Co., 1956.

Ramdas, Swami. *World is God.* Kanhangad, S. India: Anandashram, 1955.

Rowland, Beryl L. *Birds With Human Souls: A Guide To Bird Symbolism.* Knoxville: University of Tennessee Press, 1978.

Sacharow, Yogi-Raj Boris. *Das Grosse Geheiminis.* Munchen: Drie Eichen Verlag, 1954.

Samples, Bob. *The Metaphoric Mind.* Reading, Mass.: Addison-Wesley Publishing Co., 1978. p. 156-176.

The Satapatha Brahmana. Vol. 41 of *Sacred Books of the East.* 1894. Reprint. Delhi: Motilal Banarsidass, 1979.

Saunders, E. Dale. *Mudra: A Study of Symbolic Gestures in Japanese Buddhist Sculpture.* Bollingen Series 58. Pantheon Books, 1960.

Schaller, George B. "Life with the King of Beasts." *National Geographic,* 135 (April 1964): 494-519.

Schultz, Jack C. "Tree tactics." *Natural History,* May, 1983.

Siegel, Lee. *Sacred and Profane Dimensions of Love In Indian Traditions as Exemplified in the Gitagovinda of Jayadeva.* London: Oxford University Press, 1978.

Simonton, O. C. *Getting Well Again.* Los Angeles: J. P. Tarcher, 1978.

The Siva Samhita. Translated by Sris Chandra Vasu. 3d ed. New Delhi: Oriental Books Reprint Corp., 1979.

Sivananda Radha, Swami. *The Divine Light Invocation*. rev. ed. Porthill, Idaho: Timeless Books, 1987.

——. *Kundalini: Yoga for the West*. Porthill, Idaho: Timeless Books, 1978.

—— *Mantras: Words of Power*. 1980. Reprint. Porthill, Idaho: Timeless Books, 1987.

Sivananda Saraswati, Swami. *Guru and Disciple*. Rishikesh, India: Yoga-Vedanta Forest University, 1955.

——. *Japa Yoga*. Rishikesh, India: Divine Life Society, 1967.

——. *The Practice of Brahmacharya*. 8th ed. Rishikesh, India: Divine Life Society, 1980.

——. *Yoga Asanas*. 12th ed. Rishikesh, India: Divine Life Society, 1962.

Tagore, Rabin I. *One Hundred Poems of Kali*. New York: Macmillan, 1961.

Taimni, I. K. *The Science of Yoga*. Wheaton, Ill.: Theosophical Publishing House, 1961.

The Thirteen Principal Upanishads. Translated by Robert E. Hume. 2d ed. rev. London: Oxford University Press, 1931.

Thirty Minor Upanishads. Translated by K. Narayanasvami Aiyar. 1914. Reprint. El Reno, Okla.: Santarasa Publications, 1980.

Tripura Rahasya or the Mystery Beyond the Trinity. Translated by Munagala S. Venkataramaiah. 2d ed. Tiruvannamalai, India: Sri Ramanasramam, 1962.

Tyberg, Judith. *Language of the Gods*. 2d ed. Los Angeles: East-West Cultural Centre, 1976.

Venkatesananda, Swami. *The Gospel of God-Love*. Divine Life Society, 1970.

——. *Yoga*. 3d ed. rev. Cape Province, S. A.: Chiltern Yoga Trust, 1971.

Vivekananda, Swami. *Karma Yoga*. Reprint. Mayavati, India: Advaita Ashrama, 1978.

——. *Raja Yoga*. Calcutta: Advaita Ashrama, 1970.

Waddell, L. Austine. *Tibetan Buddhism*. 1895. Reprint. Dover Publications, 1972.

Walsh, Roger N. and Frances Vaughan. *Beyond Ego: Transpersonal Dimensions in Psychology*. Los Angeles: J. P. Tarcher, 1980.

Watts, Alan U. *Nature, Man and Woman*. New York: Pantheon Books, 1958.

Went, Frits W. *The Plants*. rev. ed. New York: Time-Life Books, 1971.

Williams, C. A. S. *Outlines of Chinese Symbolism and Art Motives*. 3d rev. ed. Rutland, Vt.: Charles E. Tuttle Co., 1974.

Wilson, Edward O. *On Human Nature*. Cambridge: Harvard University Press, 1978.

Wood, Ernest. *Practical Yoga Ancient and Modern*. 1948. Reprint. Hollywood, Calif.: Wilshire Book Co., 1976.

Zimmer, Heinrich. *Myths and Symbols in Indian Art and Civilization*. Edited by Joseph Campbell. Bollingen Series 6. 1946. Reprint. Princeton: Princeton University Press, 1972.

————. *Philosophies of India*. Bollingen Series 26. New York: Pantheon Books, 1951.

index

interconnectedness of all life 59
    see also dependence
interdependence 6, 13, 14, 59
intuition xviii, 45, 109
Iran 151
Islam 94, 151
Iyengar, B.K.S. 6, 8, 65, 267,
    272

J

Jesus Christ 61, 113, 177, 186,
    222, 272-273, 283
Jewish legends and traditions
    138, 194
jiva 43
John, the Evangelist 203, 283
Judeo-Christian tradition 150
Jungian psychology 203
Juno 193
Jupiter 218

K

Kabbalah 111
Kailasa Mountain 36
Kali, the Hindu goddess 242
Kaliya, the cobra 156
Kama, the Hindu god 94, 97
Krishna, 95, 96, 126, 150, 156,
    193, 234
Kukkutasana 182-189
Kundalini
    serpent 246
    Shakti 156
    system 5, 12, 13, 138, 177,
    270
    Yoga xviii, 281
Kurmasana 160-173
Kuvalayananda, Swami 7-8
Kwan Yin, the Chinese goddess
    178, 193

L

Lakhmu and Lakhamu, the
    Babylonian god and goddess
    151
Lakshmi, the Hindu goddess
    155, 193
language 12-14, 59, 218, 284,
    285
Liberation 46, 125, 268
Light 8, 11, 47, 97, 113, 124,
    126, 142, 196, 222, 247, 260,
    273
limitations 95
lion 283
lion posture 238-249
listening 74, 222
logic 44
lotus posture 118-129
love 55, 61, 94, 97, 196, 269
    erotic 126

M

male, masculine 83, 96, 107,
    151, 178, 186, 267
man 166, 268
manipulation 15, 74
Manipura Chakra, see chakra
Mantra 5, 13, 48, 97, 164, 287
Manu 139
Mark, the Evangelist 245, 283
Mars 185
Maslow, Abraham 9
Matsyasana 132-145
Matthew, Saint 283
Mayurasana 190-197
meditation 32, 60, 125, 164, 167,
    170, 223, 256, 287
Medusa, the Greek gorgon 153
Mesopotamians 137
Mexico 202

sweetness in 94
as a teacher 17
Parvati 272
Paschimottanasana 64-69, 95
Paul, Saint 259
peacock posture 190-197
personality aspects 9, 16-18, 87,
  96, 274, 281
  changes in 76
  conflicting 9
  greedy 108
  identification of 167
  interfering 258
  opinions and beliefs of 281
  symbol in the Gita 268
  transcending 9, 13, 17, 273,
  280
perspective 74
phoenix 194, 195, 223
Pisces 138
plough posture 80-89, 281
polarity 3-4, 35
prana 48, 49, 62, 168
prayer 60, 61, 164
pride 73, 187, 193
prophecy 166
protection 165
psychoanalysis 274
psychology 279-280
Pudicita (symbol) 166

R

Ra, the Egyptian god 105, 151,
  166, 201
Radha 126
rainbow (symbol) 94, 97, 151
Ramachandra 95
Ramakrishna 36, 219, 231
Rank, Otto 11
reason 44, 109
rebirth, reincarnation 151, 194

reflection xvii, 13, 14, 18-19, 32,
  60, 107, 140, 167, 170, 279
relaxation 95, 256, 259
renunciation 11, 84, 125, 126
resistance 257
responsibility 15, 16, 19, 44, 46,
  53, 268
rest 260
resurrection 157, 194, 196
Rishis 284, 285, 288
Romans, Roman mythology 59,
  151, 166, 186, 192, 217

S

sacrifice 138, 223
sadhana 279-281
Salamba Sarvangasana 50-55
Salamba Shirshasana 40-49
Sarada Devi 219
Saraswati, the Hindu goddess
  126, 193
Satchitananda 11, 62
Scandinavia 106, 113, 186, 202
scorpion 259
scorpion posture 174-179
security 43, 83
self-analysis 17
self-glorification 177
self-gratification 75, 85
self-image 21
self-importance 10, 53, 106, 171,
  178
selfishness 10, 152
self-justification 74
selfless service 10-11
self-mastery xviii
self-observation 21, 274
Self-recognition 274
self-will 17, 53, 55, 83, 96, 152
self-worth 16
Selket, the Egyptian goddess 177